School Safety

School Safety

One Cheeseburger at a Time

Susan T. Vickers and Kevin L. Smith

To Tameka

Kevin Smith

Susan Vickers ☺

ROWMAN & LITTLEFIELD

Lanham • Boulder • New York • London
Copublished with AASA

Published by Rowman & Littlefield
An imprint of The Rowman & Littlefield Publishing Group, Inc.
4501 Forbes Boulevard, Suite 200, Lanham, Maryland 20706
www.rowman.com

6 Tinworth Street, London SE11 5AL, United Kingdom

British Library Cataloguing in Publication Information Available

Library of Congress Cataloging-in-Publication Data Available

ISBN 978-1-4758-5313-1 (cloth : alk. paper)
ISBN 978-1-4758-5314-8 (pbk. : alk. paper)
ISBN 978-1-4758-5315-5 (electronic)

∞™ The paper used in this publication meets the minimum requirements of American National Standard for Information Sciences—Permanence of Paper for Printed Library Materials, ANSI/NISO Z39.48-1992.

Contents

Foreword

It is always interesting how the intersection of lives impacts those around us. It was through some impromptu events orchestrated by Technical Sergeant Vedder of the New York State Police that Dr. Susan T. Vickers and Dr. Kevin L. Smith became acquaintances and then friends (see Acknowledgment). It was through their professional friendship when they worked together to help teach school employees about the various facets of school safety, both physical and mental, that the premise for this book commenced.

Dr. Vickers had previously written an article for the New York State School Boards Association, OnBoard magazine in September 2018, entitled "As Educational Leaders We Must Become Security Experts." Following this article she wrote another article in April 2019 entitled "Educational Leader and Security Professional" for the School Administrator magazine of the American Association of School Administrators (AASA). The topic of school safety and security is an issue that Dr. Vickers lives with daily being a superintendent of a school district. The safety and well-being of all her students and staff remains a priority for her. This book was written to help school leaders navigate the requirements and lessons learned from past incidents to prevent their repetition in their own schools.

Dr. Kevin L. Smith is Distinguished Life Fellow of the American Psychiatric Association. He trained at Walter Reed National Military Hospital in internal medicine, neurology, and psychiatry, and served as chief resident in his senior year. He is Board Certified in General and Forensic Psychiatry. Over the 40 years of his military and civilian careers, Dr. Smith has focused on assessing dangerousness risk. He has evaluated hundreds of murderers and violent criminals and testified at their trials.

In the 1980s, U.S. Army European Command called upon Dr. Smith's knowledge and experience in dangerousness risk when an epidemic of suicides occurred. This was the beginning of SAD PERSONS, which is one of the major prevention lessons that permeate this book. In 1985 and within one year of implementing this training program with all active duty military members and Department of Defense Dependents Schools (DODDS) staff and educators, the suicide epidemic stopped and even accidental deaths dropped dramatically. Dr. Smith received the Meritorious Service Medal for his SAD PERSONS initiative.

Dr. Smith has been called upon to provide trainings and consultations to the Association of Justices of the Supreme Court of the State of New York, the Department of Homeland and Emergency Services, the FBI, the CIA, the DC SWAT, the Secret Services, the U.S. Coast Guard, the New York and New Jersey Port Authority, the New York State Bridge Authority, the New York State Police, West Point, school districts and numerous local law enforcement agencies and Police Chiefs Associations to provide dangerousness risk assessment trainings and to assist with active scenes requiring dangerousness risk assessments. Of all the numerous awards the doctor has received in his career, he is most proud of being the recipient of the New York State Senate Resolution No. 4214 honoring him with the Meritorious Citizenship Award for Justice, for which the Police Chiefs Association nominated him.

That chance meeting with Dr. Vickers a few years ago led Dr. Kevin L. Smith to this team effort to write a book that covers the main aspects of school safety and security. Logistics of how to protect a school, combined with the strategy of how to keep people safe are the main points that flow throughout the chapters. School safety is not just about having school resource officers and reporting mechanisms for instances of bullying. It is so much more than that. It takes time, commitment to physical and mental resources, and the vision of having a safe and nurturing school environment.

Acknowledgment

This book was made possible by the passionate and persistent professionalism and dedicated work of New York State Trooper Craig Vedder.

Trooper Vedder's commitment to protecting schools and their communities made quite an impression on both Dr. Vickers and Dr. Smith. Dr. Vickers requested that Trooper Vedder come and speak with both the students and the staff at her school. His message was well received, and as such he was asked back on more than one occasion to speak about school safety. When planning for a conference day focused on school safety, Trooper Vedder was chosen to lead a panel discussion. He was ecstatic when his personal mentor on this topic, Dr. Smith, was available to join him for the conference day. The training on this spring day, as well as Trooper Vedder's and Dr. Smith's impact on the school district, have led to both numerous safety and security changes as well as a new normal. As a result of this relationship, Dr. Smith and Trooper Vedder have traveled across New York State presenting to schools, law enforcement organizations, and key New York State Police Leaders. The message is clear, concise, and very timely. And through this book, it is now available to everyone.

In 2017, the Police Chiefs Association honored Trooper Vedder's service excellence with the Meritorious Police Service Award—Community Service. Specifically, it was Sgt. Vedder's excellent performance record and his active and sustained involvement with preventing a nine-year-old boy's suicide that brought him the special attention of his superiors. In the case of the suicidal boy, he worked closely with the school's assistant superintendent, local police, first responders, mobile mental health, social services, and the child's family to ensure they were getting the support that they needed. Throughout this tense situation, Trooper Vedder demonstrated his professional training and demeanor, constantly reassessing and reviewing prior decisions, and

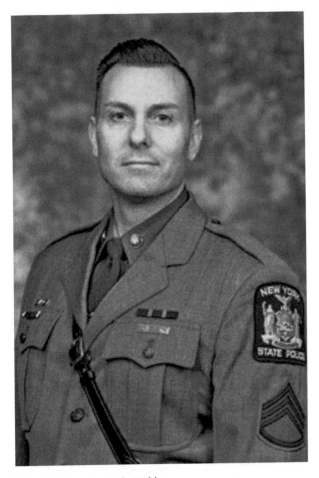

Image A.1   Technical Sergeant Craig Vedder.

appropriately addressing the emotional needs and safety concerns of other
involved stakeholders. Trooper Vedder's professional and methodical intervention in this case was instrumental in ensuring the safety of the student's
parents, and also securing the safety and well-being of the nine-year-old student and everyone at his school. Furthermore, his actions provided a nexus
to treatment for the child. Were it not for his actions, this case may very well
have had a tragic ending. His highly creditable actions in this case were honored with the Meritorious Police Service—Community Service award.

Soon thereafter, and much to the chagrin of Dr. Vickers and Dr. Smith,
Trooper Vedder was promoted as Technical Sergeant at the New York State
Division Headquarters in Albany. There he has several important respon-
sibilities, including oversight of the New York State Police School and

Community Outreach Program, as well as interfacing with other New York State agencies on safety and security issues, such as the Department of Education, Department of Homeland Security and Emergency Services, and the Department of Health.

We are all honored and safer due to Technical Sergeant Craig Vedder's dedicated and professional law enforcement commitment. We thank you, Technical Sergeant Craig Vedder!

Respectfully and with sincere appreciation,
Susan T. Vickers, EdD, and Kevin L. Smith, MD

Introduction

It is not the likeliness of a dangerous event occurring that moves us to prevent it, but rather it is the raw evilness of these incidents that compels us to act.

"Shots fired at a local school. Injured and dead confirmed by local police." Hearing this breaking news is akin to getting punched in the stomach. For the moment it is hard to breathe and incomprehensible how this could possibly have occurred, yet again.

Next the mind races to the expected fallout. This incident will dominate the media for the next few weeks. Interviews of anyone and everyone near the attack will be aired and published by all media networks.

Following will be the diatribe from each political party as they try to sway public opinion toward their political agendas. The list of those injured and killed will give way to political debate with jabs thrown across each aisle. More gun control will be argued for, more background checks, lobbying for more money for mental health will be center stage, and there will be questioning if the school did all they could to protect students and staff.

The final funeral will be held and the last interview aired. Lastly, the memorial flowers, now dead, will be removed. But the story does not, and should not, end there.

For most of the nation, after the news ebbs, a sense of hope will develop. Another dawn brings renewed hope, and with this school doors will open with the routine that existed before the chaos of the school shooting. All appears promising. That is, for everyone except school leaders.

Active attacks on schools and social entities are emotionally draining and devastating acts that terrorize the very soul of America. Criminal acts of

violence far too often get tweeted about or show up on social media, to the
point where it is almost a typical daily occurrence.

In the two weeks following the February 14, 2018, shooting in Parkland,
Florida, at Marjory Stoneman Douglas High School, there were forty school
shootings and violent threats made in Upstate New York. Copycats plagued
schools nationwide. Parents demanded to know how the district leadership
was going to protect their children.

Unfortunately, the answer is that school leaders are no better prepared than
the average citizen. However, all the District-Wide School Safety plans and
Building-Level Emergency Response Plans are filed with the state. These
plans address the systems approach to who reports to whom in the perfectly
executed scenario, but lack the fine details for how to prevent, act, and refine
all the facets included in school safety and security.

Numerous articles, white papers, and seminars are offered annually to help
make schools safer with a lot of the work and expectations for action pressed
upon school leaders. What is lacking is a cohesive plan from either the state
or the federal departments of education. School and student safety are a
district-level decision. School leaders need to absorb as much information
as possible on the options available to them, in a cost-effective manner, and
implement a safety and security plan with integrity and fidelity.

What is not conveyed is the consequence and impact this has on school
leaders who entered into a profession with a focus on student learning in
order to prepare our leaders and citizens of tomorrow. What they now face
is a new dimension of their job description. #SchoolleaderSecurityProfes-
sional—an interesting expectation that is held in communities across the
nation in regard to their school leaders. What many community members may
not be aware of is the cold hard fact that no one in school administration has
had formal training in school safety or security.

School leaders are vested in education, as most come from the teaching
and counseling ranks. To become a certified school administrator, they have
studied and earned a Certificate of Advanced Study from an accredited college. Their coursework includes a litany of classes such as those identified
in table I.1.

The list of possible courses is extensive. However, not one of these courses
addresses safety and security, or prepares leaders for the task of preventing
school violence, nor does it provide them with the knowledge of how to
secure a school while at the same time ensuring a nurturing school environment. There is no preparation except for that which is gleaned from reading
articles or attending reactive seminars, and yet the expectation for performance is on par with academic growth.

The New York State Education Department (NYSED) in accordance
with the school emergency response planning legislation requires all public

Table I.1 Required College Courses for School Administrators (General Representation)

Principles of Financial Leadership	Educational Leadership and the Law
Principles of Curriculum Leadership	Strategic Supervision and Leadership
Principles of Organizational Leadership	Special Education Administration
Principal Leadership	Fundamentals of Administration
Principles of Special Education Leadership	School Principalship
School Law for Building and District Leaders	School Business Management for Building and District Leaders
Curriculum Theory	School Personnel Management for Building and District Leaders
Leadership for Diverse Learners and Communities	Supervision: Improvement of Instruction for Building and District Leaders
Leadership for Literacy Development	Administrative Internship

Self-designed.

schools to submit their District-Wide School Safety plans and Building-Level Emergency Response Plans each school year. The New York State Schools Against Violence in Education (SAVE) Act, enacted in 2000, was developed in an effort to increase school safety in New York's public schools. A template for entering the information is utilized to ensure uniformity. Here is where the uniformity ends.

School districts in New York State are required by law to submit their School Safety Plan (Building and District plans) annually, but integrity and fidelity of this action have fallen short of expectations. The NYS comptroller completed a spot check in 2019 of the School Safety requirements for 14 school districts and found only half completed the requirement to submit the plans to local policing agencies.

On a positive note, 99% have shared their plans with the state police (Randall, 2019). Policing agencies are required to receive the same District-Wide School Safety plans and Building-Level Emergency Response Plans each school year. A file is received electronically from each public school in their jurisdiction. Is there a requirement that law enforcement review and train with these documents? What is the requirement(s) for coordination with the schools? Whose job is it to ensure such collaborative work occurs? To date, this coordination is addressed at the local level by both school leaders and policing agencies.

The audit by the NYS comptroller did not find consistency with the SAVE Act legislation across the state. Does the lack of consistency with document filing across the state equate to unsafe schools, or does this mean schools are working as independent contractors as they seek safe and secure school buildings? The answer is not an easy yes or no as there appears to be a myriad of action taking place to ensure secure and safe schools.

Training for students and staff, akin to fire drills, lockdowns, lockouts, stay in place, and evacuation are mandated each year. There is a good reason to practice drilling on where to go and what to do when an emergency is called. The questions are: How is the emergency called? Is it "code red," "lockdown," or "level one"? Do first responders know all the names? Who updates any changes and provides the training? Many questions and the answers are beginning to take shape.

Where then is the much-needed action plan? Given the epidemic of school violence over the past few years, it is clearly evident that schools are a premier soft target. Schools are built to be nurturing environments where everyone gets a second, third, or fourth chance. The goal is to ensure everyone who graduates is an active citizen and has the wherewithal to successfully enter the workforce or college. With limitless chances, little information on how to make schools safe without creating cold institutions, the question of how to create a long-term plan is a quagmire. Balancing warm and caring with state-of-the-art protection from vicious attacks appears contradictory.

Nurturing versus state-of-the-art protection is dichotomous. Or is it? Does it have to be one or the other? If not, how then do schools and boards of education step in to create a balanced environment that completely protects students and staff while making it nurturing to the point that the students and staff are unaware of the armed fortress around them?

Learn. Develop. Implement. Three simple steps. Ah, not so simple. Whereas schools may act as microcosms of society, they do interact with the public at large. Specifically, in regard to local law enforcement, school districts need to create a symbiotic relationship. If all schools created their own safety and security plans imagine the nightmare that would cause for first responders. Common protocols, language, and plans need to be in place, practiced, and drilled until they are as routine as a fire drill.

This book does not profess to have all the answers; rather, it is written to help everyone guide their thinking as it relates to school safety and security in the twenty-first century. It offers a comprehensive overview of violence to highlight the historical and current issue as it impacts schools and our communities. Additionally, a correlation between school violence and mental health issues are addressed as they are inexplicably intertwined. Takeaways from active shooter training, threat assessments, and dangerousness risk assessments provide proactive and tangible steps that school leaders can utilize immediately. Finally, real-life case studies are presented to illustrate the implementation of the strategies at our disposal to various sites and situations in order to help prevent a continuance of these issues.

The overall goal is to prevent the next attack from happening, or at the very least contain the injuries. Columbine shocked the world, and at Sandy Hook and Parkland we vowed never to let this happen again. To date schools and policing agencies have thwarted some would-be attacks but are not at the point where school attacks are completely removed. School safety and security is a work in progress with no end point in sight.

School shootings, whether they result in injury or death, grab our attention and cause people to stop and pause. These gut-wrenching events are horrific, and at the same time they are statistically rare events. There are more car crashes and farm-related tragedies than school shootings. The chances of being struck by lightning even supersede the likelihood of being shot and killed during a school shooting. *It is not the likeliness of the event occurring that moves us to prevent such events; rather, it is the raw evilness of these incidents that compels us to act.*

Chapter 1

How Did We Get Here?

Keeping our school children safe requires the shared commitment from states, school leaders, and communities.

It all began on November 12, 1840, in Charlottesville, Virginia, when Joseph Semmes shot his law professor, John Anthony Gardner Davis. Professor Davis died 3 days later from his wounds. In the 179-year time span since that shooting, there have been approximately 603 total school shootings, or an average of 3.4 per year. This number includes shootings on school buses and the discharge of firearms on school property.

Another major school shooting that shocked the nation occurred 126 years later, on August 1, 1966, when a sniper shot and killed 17 people at the University of Texas. The sniper positioned himself in a clock tower and used that location to easily fire upon innocent people. This event is eerily similar to the October 2017 shooting at the Route 91 Music Festival in Las Vegas, where a determined gunman, a prime location, and no one questioning his habits prior to the shooting resulted in the deaths of 58 people and left another 413 wounded.

Why schools? Why concerts or open-air markets? The answers are quite simple: each presents a target-rich environment that is often soft on safety and security, and each is often perceived by the perpetrator as having caused them a significant real or imagined grievance that formed the basis for their profound resentment. An emotional significance to the shooter of the physical layout, combined with mental distress, heightens their propensity for violent action.

After each atrocity the question on the minds of the survivors and those watching via their smartphone or TV is why no one saw it coming. As shocking as it may sound, many people do bear witness to the planning stages;

their minds are just not programmed to view the isolated planning acts as those of a killer. Generally, family, friends, and coworkers are able to assist investigators in gathering information to help them learn about the cause of the shooting incidents.

In retrospect, we put the pieces together. Much like a Monday morning quarterback, who picks apart the weekend's game to determine how the team could have won, hindsight with school shooting incidents is also 20/20. But if we only look back and do not look to the future, we will be forever doomed to recapitulate the paradigm.

Those who do not learn history are doomed to repeat it. Adolf Hitler wrote in *Mein Kampf* about his plan to eliminate the Jewish population and to bring glory and power back to Germany. The Columbine shooters made a video for one of their classes depicting exactly what they were going to do. They were inspired by the 1995 release of the movie *The Basketball Diaries*, starring Leonardo DiCaprio. Adam Lanza, from the Sandy Hook shooting, wrote online to a fellow gamer that he incessantly felt nothing other than scorn for humanity. Here is my plan, what are you going to do about it? Disbelief? Fear? Is it a joke? That no one acted upon these proliferations of devastation is frustrating. The human race learns and adapts and this is where we have stagnated. We are adapting, but doing so as individual contractors with lack of cohesiveness and urgency.

No longer is it acceptable to make comments that 20 years earlier were met with benign reactions. "I am so mad that I could just kill you," is an example of a statement that 20 years ago may have been met with a quick retort, but today results in calls to mental health workers and law enforcement.

Active attacks on schools and social entities are emotionally draining and devastating acts that terrorize the very soul of American communities. Criminal acts of violence far too often get tweeted about or show up on Facebook, to the point where it is almost a typical daily occurrence. God help us all if we ever get to the point where this type of news does not cause a gut-wrenching reaction.

What, then, is the long-term plan of action? Numerous articles, white papers, and seminars are offered to help make schools safer with a lot of the work and expectation for action pressed upon school leaders. These school leaders are vested in education, as most come from the teaching and counseling ranks.

In May 2019 the Johns Hopkins University announced it will be creating short courses to educate school leaders on the standards for school safety. The push for this type of education has grown in urgency with the Sandy Hook massacre in December 2012. The Center for Safe and Healthy Schools is still in the planning stages, but they have already indicated the trifecta of topics to be addressed: trauma, bullying, and gun violence.

Johns Hopkins University has not indicated when the courses will be up and running, but the writing on the wall is clear: there will be community representation, educators, school leaders, and policy makers enrolling in the courses. Utilizing the research capabilities associated with the university, this center will address the cognitive mental acuity necessary for school leaders to keep students healthy, the community engaged, and the schools safe and secure from threats.

Until such a program is up and running throughout the nation with integrity and fidelity, the only other preparation available is that which is gleaned from reading articles, white papers, or attending seminars. However, the overwhelming expectation for safety and security is on par with academic growth and achievement. Some of the documentation available to assist school leaders is excellent and should serve as the foundation for all school safety and security models.

The School Safety and Security Council (SSSC) issued a white paper in 2016 entitled "Active Shooter." This document serves as a foundational guide for the prevention of active shooter incidents. In July 2018, the U.S. Department of Secret Service National Threat Assessment Center (NTAC) issued an "Enhancing School Safety Using a Threat Assessment Model" paper to serve as an operational guide for preventing targeted school violence. Prior to this release the U.S. Department of Homeland Security released a paper in February 2018 entitled "Making Schools Safer." It is not surprising to see such a strong hand from the government in this field as school shooters have much in common with terrorists.

Whereas many safety publications from the federal government have been released, none was sent directly to school superintendents, or school leaders, although it is clear through the language presented that they were part of the intended audience. Thus, school leaders need to search for these types of sources and information as some are excellent tools for helping to prevent violence within their districts. School leaders have a full plate of state and federal mandates and reporting on top of the day-to-day issues associated with leading and managing a school district. Not providing federal or state documents directly to all school leaders across the nation is frustrating. How can they provide for safety and security when the professionals are not playing nice in the sandbox by sharing with all major stakeholders?

Who is to blame, or is no one to blame? Quite possibly a new position within the Federal Department of Education should be created that is responsible for vetting and then sharing information as well as procedures among all state departments of education. In turn the states can create policy and regulations that will enhance uniformity and oversight of school safety and security. As it currently exists, there is a lot of activity taking place, but without a concrete vision that is clearly articulated to all stakeholders, the energy is being lost. The destination is not being achieved as the path to get there is muddied and mired in a myriad of suggestions.

Randolf D. Alles, director of the U.S. Secret Service, included a message in the introduction to "Enhancing School Safety Using a Threat Assessment Model" operational guide, that specifically notes the need to provide updated research and guidance to school personnel, law enforcement, and other public safety partners. The question now is how this information gets uniformly shared, adopted, and implemented with integrity and fidelity. If this manual becomes shelf art the effort behind a valuable document that is directly targeted toward providing school safety will be lost.

Law enforcement personnel are generally not in attendance at school leadership conferences. Conversely, neither are school leaders at conferences geared for law enforcement. Hoping that the information presented at such conferences and trainings will permeate to all other key stakeholders, even those not invited, is inadequate. The U.S. Department of Education in cooperation with the Department of Education in each U.S. state needs to work in coordination with agencies such as the Secret Service to ensure a uniform model and language is implemented. Anything less places school children and staff in jeopardy as they become possible targets of the next school shooting.

School shootings, although on the rise, are not at an epidemic proportion as some media outlets would lead the public to believe. With the advent of social media and the proprietary rights for cable news, society by and large is aware of a situation in today's world as the event is still unfolding. No longer do we wait with bated breath for the evening news. Consequently, not only are we now made more aware of issues occurring across the nation, but we are also given much more depth of information than was available a few decades ago when this trend was in its infancy.

A few weeks after attending a seminar that addressed how to enact a dangerousness risk assessment (DRA), an assistant school superintendent was called upon to do just that. Prior to the incident that was about to face the assistant superintendent, 3 young boys committed suicide, and now a fourth student was on the precipice of duplicating the act. On the spot, the assistant superintendent enacted what she had learned at the seminar and phoned the forensic psychiatrist for support. Thankfully, due to her knowledge of DRAs, the assistant superintendent prevented the suicide and helped the young man get the counseling he needed.

America is beginning to take notice and in turn is taking action. By attending a seminar on school safety this assistant superintendent was able to save the life of a young man that was about to end tragically. Imagine the impact if all school leaders received the same training.

There are definite signs and symptoms of increasing potential for dangerous behavior in all of us. First and foremost, we must keep in the forefront of our minds: "Hurt people hurt people!" No one just steps out of their bedroom one day and resolves, "Today I'm going to kill 24 random grade-school children with an automatic assault rifle." There will be an emerging and growing perceived grievance that precipitates resentments that can be identified.

That said, however, no one can accurately predict or even postdict violent behavior. In fact, the very person who has planned out their assault precisely and specifically cannot truly predict their own violence, because things can change at any moment. They may need or choose to abandon Plan A and deploy Plan B instead, or even create a new Plan C. Therefore, predicting violence is entirely off the table.

There are very basic, practical signs and symptoms when an individual is developing an increased risk of behaving dangerously, to which we can respond in safe and effective ways to reduce or even eliminate their elevated risk. This is DRA.

KEY IDEAS TO REMEMBER

School shootings are not a twenty-first-century phenomenon. Rather, they have been an issue since 1840. What is new is the fact that these events are now broadcast around the world in real-time, so that everyone is exposed to the fear and panic as it is occurring. This makes it more than a human interest story. This makes it personal.

Soft targets such as schools, open-air markets, and concerts draw the attention of active shooters, but not because of the ease the target represents. There is an emotional significance to the target for the shooter, and when this is combined with mental distress the propensity for violence is heightened.

The U.S. Secret Service NTAC, the SSSC, and the U.S. Department of Homeland Security have issued guidance on how to stop school shootings. In doing so they offer a litany of processes and procedures that, if implemented, should be able to thwart would-be attackers and get them the mental health help they need. One fact is certain concerning why this is happening: *Hurt people, hurt people*!

Chapter 2

Actions Speak Louder than Words

It took some students in Parkland, Florida, to stand up for reform and change after the deadly shooting at Marjory Stoneman Douglas High School.

The last fire that occurred in a school that resulted in death occurred in 1958. Prior to the publication of this book, the last time students were shot and killed while at school was on a Thursday, November 14, 2019, in Santa Clarita, California. By the time you read this book, there will likely be several more. In 2019 alone, there were 14 school shootings that resulted in 4 deaths and 23 injuries. In 2018 there were 24 school shootings with 35 deaths and 79 injuries. By this account, 2019 was a better year as there were fewer shootings, and yet schools still continue to experience these tragic events.

Actions speak louder than words, and thankfully both word and action are combining in an effort to lessen school shootings. Action is found in a three-pronged plan of action as referenced in figure 2.1.

On September 13, 2010, the Dignity for All Students Act (DASA) was signed into law in New York State. DASA specifically ensured the right of all children to attend school in a safe, welcoming, and caring environment. It was the state's attempt to curb the tide of bullying for all students. It prohibits the harassment and discrimination of students by students and by school personnel. Every public school was required to amend their Code of Conduct to reflect the prohibition of discrimination and harassment of students by students or staff in age-appropriate language. All schools in receipt of state funding are required to have annual DASA training for all staff, and each school district must have at least one DASA Coordinator per building. These efforts are in place to ensure everyone is aware of the law and the reporting requirements.

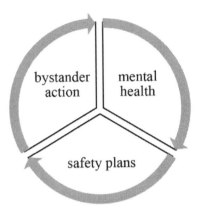

Figure 2.1   3-Prong Actions to Lessen Violence in Schools. *Source*: Self-Designed.

The New York State Education Department (NYSED), like many education departments across the nation, established a School Safety Task Force in 2013. Through their work it was determined that school culture and student engagement, data use and reporting, and building security and infrastructure were the three areas that necessitated action. In turn, these areas became the blueprint for 36 recommendations for prekindergarten through grade 12 in New York State. Implementation of these plans was designed to occur incrementally over five years.

Reporting requirements changed with the findings and actions of the NYS School Safety Task Force. Instead of being reactive and focusing only on the discipline, the Task Force changed the reporting format to promote and measure school climate as well as development of a focus on social emotional learning (SEL). The new form is known as School Safety and Educational Climate (SSEC), and it collects data on only the most serious incidents along with school climate indicators. The goal remains consistent in its effort to end the increase of bullying in schools.

Most importantly, this Task Force began the important aspect of requiring schools to use the same safety and security language in regard to their emergency drills and plans. There are five types of emergency drills and plans for all public schools in the New York State: lockdown, lockout, shelter-in-place, hold-in-place, and evacuate. Every NYS public school now utilizes these terms for their plans and drills. Given the increase in school shootings and the fact that the last death caused by a fire in a school occurred in 1958, NYSED subsequently reduced the number of fire drills from 12 to 8 and added 4 lockdown drills per year.

Interestingly enough, these types of terrorist attacks against schools, businesses, churches, synagogues, concerts, and shopping malls have added new common vocabulary across the country. "Active shooter" and "shelter in place" do not need an explanation when broadcasted. It is now common for movie theaters, shopping malls, houses of worship, and schools to have armed guards. Having a police presence provides for some peace of mind, although these same institutions continue to practice lockdown drills to prepare everyone for the possibility of a shooter.

Drills and school resource officers serve as deterrents, but they are not foolproof. Nothing is foolproof in regards to preventing an active shooter. NYSED's Task Force acknowledged this and developed a tool for measuring school climate with a focus on the SEL of all students.

One commonality woven into every active shooter incident since the first shot rang out from the clock tower at the University of Texas in 1966 is that each shooter developed a plan and had communicated the plan, in whole or in part, to someone well before the event. Hindsight is informative, and as such we have learned from each atrocity what to look for as someone is developing their plan. This knowledge finds a concerted effort by Kindergarten-12 grade schools as they begin an earnest focus on SEL in the classroom.

Berlin (2019) references the goal of SEL as to helping students learn the skills needed for managing the emotions that we feel every day along with learning coping techniques to help students through challenging emotions. Once these skills are in place the next key step is helping students to foster, develop, and maintain positive relationships. Contrary to popular opinion, it is possible to profile a school attacker. One common attribute is their perception of being bullied, isolated, and/or scorned, which subsequently evolves into grievances and resentments. The acronyms BRGR (pronounced "burger") and CBRGR (pronounced "cheeseburger") provide simple reminders of what to look for when a potential attacker is suspected, as illustrated in figure 2.2.

BRGR = Behaviors, Risk factors, Grievances, Resentments
CBRGR = Changes in Behaviors, Risk factors, Grievances, Resentments

SEL offers guidance in helping to recognize such perceptions in an effort to employ interventions to help address, and/or remove, the resentment or grievance.

In keeping with the recommendations from the Task Force, NYS Education Department developed a tool to measure school climate as an effort to target schools that may require additional support. SEL resources have been provided across the state to schools, and mental health organizations are also offering training for school districts.

Consequently, along with teaching to the standards, creating critical thinkers and civic-minded citizens, schools now need to add another layer to their daily instruction. SEL is taught by being cognizant of the impact our words and actions have in regard to what students learn.

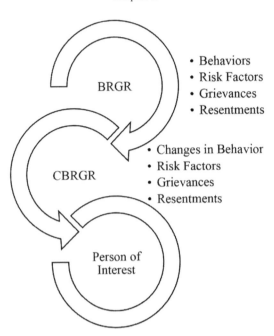

- Behaviors
- Risk Factors
- Grievances
- Resentments

- Changes in Behavior
- Risk Factors
- Grievances
- Resentments

Figure 2.2　Key Identifying Features for a Person of Interest. *Source*: Self-Designed.

Humphrey et al. (2011) propose that SEL focuses on social skills and interactions these skills have on people's ability to successfully navigate relationships. They further note that all learning is both social and emotional, and as such is something that is already part of the educational process. As noted in the name, these skills focus on social and emotional behaviors. The learning associated with this process focuses on training children to recognize their own emotions, manage their emotions, and subsequently understand the impact that their reactions have on others around them. This in turn leads to responsible decision-making, development of positive relationships, and the ability to develop a tool bag for possible actions when things are not going smoothly. These pro-social behaviors are tools that they will utilize their entire lives.

In essence, SEL is what the humanities would refer to as the soft skills in life. By teaching and modeling SEL in schools, the goal is to help children develop the wherewithal to be agents of their own learning. In keeping with this same vein of soft skill learning, for the classroom teacher and school leader, this is not so much about adding to the curriculum. Rather, SEL is about how we teach more than it is about what we teach.

When pro-social behaviors are internalized by school children, the overarching premise is that discipline issues and classroom management issues should decrease. Learning how to identify triggers and appropriate responses to them is a life skill that is applicable to a wide range of situations. This is a dynamic process that begins in toddlers and continues throughout our lives. Developing the ability to control how you react to what confronts you, empathize for what those around you are experiencing, and know that you always have options is the goal of SEL. If purposefully implemented throughout school, at all levels, students should be able to develop self-confidence and improve their overall self-efficacy.

Given the simplistic design of SEL, the idea of building the soft skills associated with social and emotional well-being, it is easy to understand why it was not prioritized in kindergarten through grade 12 (K-12) education until recently. Previously, the goal of education focused on the "three R's": reading, writing, and arithmetic. Over all the years these categories have grown immensely to include much more rigorous standards and curriculum, but the premise of focusing on academics morphed. Character education which was woven into curriculum is now replaced by a more specific language known as SEL. SEL is woven into all subject areas as a language and foundation and not a stand-alone subject. This holistic approach is supported by research in terms of its ability to take hold and help the development of pro-social behaviors in children.

The soft skills of learning about emotions and behaviors appear to have taken a more subtle approach in that they dominate the themes of children's books. Bedtime stories and other children's literature focus on friendships, sharing, caring, empathy, tolerance, diversity, and the like. Children were being exposed to SEL through this genre, even if the intention was not to develop these skills, but instead to tell them a good story.

So, what happened? Why is there an uptick in school violence, and why are the messages in these children's books not being retained?

The University of Texas shooting in 1966 shocked the nation as it was reported on the nightly news programming and front-page headlines of the newspapers. Columbine made the nation sit up and take notice with the live reports from outside the school. As a nation we grieved the senseless loss of life. School leaders, teachers, and community members empathized while secretly reassuring themselves that it would not happen in their school district. Unfortunately, it continued and when the atrocity occurred on December 14, 2012, at the Sandy Hook Elementary School in Newtown, Connecticut, the nation was mortified. Images of tiny coffins made the strongest of us break. Demands for action rang out loud and clear throughout the nation.

There have been over 2,000 mass shootings in the United States since the Sandy Hook shooting where 20 students and 6 adults lost their lives. Before any major changes could occur to stem the tide of these acts of violence, the advent of twenty-first-century technology ripped at our hearts, minds, and souls. We bore witness to shootings as they were unfolding through live video thanks to twenty-first-century technology.

Fifty people were killed at a nightclub in Orlando, Florida, on June 12, 2016. This was the deadliest mass shooting in modern America until a little over a year later, when a gunman opened fire from a hotel room in Las Vegas on attendees at a music festival. This tragedy killed 59 people and assumed the title of the deadliest attack in modern American history. This shooting was streamed on social media and the world bore witness to raw fear, death, and darkness.

Scenes of children and adults running and screaming for their lives still send a chill down our spines. What no longer remains is the thought that it cannot happen here. No state in the union is without its own story of tragedy. The fear is that someday we may become desensitized to such criminal acts.

It took some students in Parkland, Florida, to stand up for reform and change after the deadly shooting on Valentine's Day in 2018 at Marjory Stoneman Douglas High School. A sense of urgency finally took hold in Florida and across the nation. School Security is now a $3 billion industry. We, as a nation, have finally begun to take a stand. State legislators and congress are setting aside money to be used for school security and safety. Mental health initiatives are finally getting funded and shared around the nation. These are small steps in the right direction.

The new normal for schools is a combination of proactive action and changes to safety and security action as well as a complete reversal in action for first responders. What was learned in regard to responding to mass shootings began with the Columbine High School shootings where a teacher bled out waiting for help. Instead of amassing out front, first responders now breach the buildings immediately.

KEY IDEAS TO REMEMBER

There is no question about it, schools function today according to a new normal that equates academics and school safety as equal priorities. In addressing this new normal, states across the nation are incorporating new programs and policy.

New York State passed the DASA in an effort to address the disrespect and bullying issue that plagued the nation. Initially, school districts reported on their DASA incidents via a reactive report that focused on how discipline was enacted. This changed as the SEL attributes were leveraged. New York State now includes incidents of student violation of the DASA elements in a report that elicits the social, emotional, and cultural climate of the school. The SSEC report is a dynamic report that provides school leaders and the state education department with real-time data concerning students and their pro-social behaviors.

Inclusive in the plan to address student behaviors are the easy-to-remember acronyms **BRGR** and **CBRGR**: burgers and cheeseburgers. Simply stated, focusing on students' behaviors, risk factors, grievances, and resentments, along with changes in these facets will allow school leaders to be proactive in addressing potential aggressors.

Lastly, there is little comfort knowing schools are on their own as they await the arrival of the first responders. Given the 3 to 5-minute expected response time frame, schools need to have plans in place that will immediately go into effect to protect the students and staff. The SSSC white paper and the documents provided by the U.S. Department of Homeland Security and the Secret Service provide steps districts need to take to maximize their internal safety and security measures during this critical time frame. Understand that your school/school district will become a victim of an aggressor. The only unknown factor is when and where.

Chapter 3

Threat Assessment in Schools

You play how you train.

None of this is rocket science. Rather, it is a new way of thinking that will help deter aggressors from trying to breach your school's entrances. There are many actions school leaders can employ without taking funding away from academics. Integrity and fidelity of implementation are the critical elements that will help develop a culture of safety and security.

There is one common statement made by law enforcement that will help school leaders sleep soundly at night: "When the call goes out that there is an active shooter at a school, we are all coming; we will be there as fast as our cars can drive, and we will remove the threat." It is our duty as school leaders to buy the first responders time to get there. Following the advice in this chapter will go a long way in meeting that goal.

It is imperative that school leaders, educators, and law enforcement understand the processes that need to be used every day to make the judgments necessary to keep the school safe and secure. Advance from 20/20 hindsight and reactive thought and move into the realm of proactive threat assessment and dangerousness risk assessment (DRA) to hone 20/20 foresight.

Threat assessment is a set plan that is reviewed annually and is implemented when a person or entity, such as a school, is facing an ongoing threat to their safety. The threat assessment plan requires ongoing reassessment of the evolving situation that will guide the decision-making process as the situation unfolds. It typically involves a multidisciplinary team that includes people that know the site and its inhabitants, multiple law enforcement agencies, emergency services, tactical emergency services, mental health personnel trained in threat assessment, the school psychologist, and so on.

Key people need to attend threat assessment, school safety, and stop the bleed trainings together. The discussions held afterward and common language will go a long way in helping to prepare and protect the school community. The U.S. Secret Service Department advocates that a threat assessment process is an effective facet for school safety. Stop the bleed training is an outgrowth of what has been learned from every shooting. Many deaths do not occur from the gunshot; rather, they occur as victims bleed out. First aid for a cut is not the same as first aid for a gunshot. Consequently, many law enforcement agencies are now adept at providing this crucial training.

The key step to thwarting a possible attack is to conduct an assessment to determine the baseline of your school's safety and security. Are your classroom doors easily breached with a simple baseball bat? Do you have a safety vestibule in each building? Do you have panic buttons and if yes, where are they located? Can every classroom phone announce a lockdown throughout the campus and dial out to access 911? The intruder will get into your building; the question is how you can best protect the children and staff until the first responders arrive. Bullet-resistant glass and solid core doors that are kept locked at all times will help to buy valuable time. Additionally, what are your school doors made of? Are the windows in your classroom doors easily breached or are they made of bullet-resistant glass?

At Columbine a 911 call included a request by the 911 agent to lock the door. The caller refused. Everyone in the room was killed as the killer came back to this room twice to fire upon the easily obtained victims. The daily operation of the school needs to include keeping all doors closed and locked throughout the day. Should an attacker get into the building, these locked doors will add an extra layer of security. Keep in mind that once faced with an anxious situation, such as a school shooter, humans will lose fine motor skills. Thus, the ability to lock the door once gunshots are heard is almost impossible to enact.

Conduct safety drills and hold safety and social-emotional discussions with both students and staff. The last fire in a school that claimed a victim was in the 1950s and the last school shooting was probably the day before you bought this book. Students need to feel empowered to come forward without fear of reprisal or disbelief. A nurturing school culture goes a long way in establishing this empowerment. Once empowered to inform school leaders of behaviors that they find unnerving the protocols can be implemented sooner to prevent another school shooting.

Through social-emotional discussions with students the threat assessment team will have the ability to see the school landscape through the eyes of their students. Ensure that the people on the team have the purview and authority to act when needed. Prevention is the optimal goal for all school leaders, teachers, parents, and students. They are all in this together as one school community.

The following list includes steps school threat assessment teams (STAT) can implement immediately to improve school safety:

1. Active shooter training needs to occur in each building in your district. After such a training at an elementary school one of the teachers stated the following:

    > You know, we practice these lockdown drills all the time. I review the stuff with my students, and I've been known to complain that we need to spend more time on academics than this stuff. Today my perspective changed, and this wasn't even real. Having to actually put into place what we discussed was nerve wracking. We need to do this every year and we need to do it in each building.

    Unsolicited advocacy from a teacher who is also a parent of elementary children further solidifies the need to practice and drill, drill, drill. We play how we train, so we have to train as if it were real. It takes time and planning, but you will find that the policing agencies in your school districts are equally nervous and determined to protect you. They need access as much as we need training.

2. Be sure to plan time for teachers and staff to ask questions. Presenting and training is a large part of the security equation, but time has to be devoted to ensure internalization. In the classroom we call it checking for understanding and closure, so we need to practice what we preach with our staff.

3. Single point of entry for each building, no exceptions. This means entering and exiting for all students, all day, every day. This includes all extracurricular activities that take place after the school day ends.

4. Make sure that your school buildings have well-lit exteriors and cameras are able to view every angle of the buildings both internally and externally. Lighting and visibility are critical aspects to have in place to help prevent incidents and to help ascertain what is happening during an incident. There was a preset delay in the cameras at Marjory Stoneman Douglas High School, and this delay was significant as law enforcement had a false sense of where the shooter was located.

5. Students should never be allowed to use a teacher's key/swipe card—ever.

6. All visitors must sign in/sign out and use designated IDs. There are systems in place now that will scan licenses to inform the school personnel if the visitor has a criminal record. The sign-in process must take place in a security vestibule that is clearly controlled by the school. No one should be able to leave the vestibule until cleared by staff personnel.

7. Visitors should not be allowed to bring bags into schools. Clear plastic bags containing needed materials (baby items, etc.) are admissible. Bags are not allowed into professional sports stadiums and yet schools allow them without question. It should be more rigorous to enter a school than an NFL stadium.

8. People working the front desks and security vestibules where visitors are allowed in should be staffed by those who know the students and community well. Never staff this position with a substitute.

9. All staff must wear their ID at work at all times. Upon leaving the district, prior employees must have their IDs immediately deactivated. All visitors must wear a badge at all times while in the building. The visitor badge should never look like the regular school staff badges; rather, they should be clearly visible as a visitor. Visitor badges must have the date and time clearly depicted, and, if possible, the photo of the visitor. Never use laminated and reusable badges for visitors.

10. Enforce a zero-tolerance policy regarding joking about school shootings and mass killings. This is not a matter to be taken lightly, so all school community members must be vigilant about this. Every school shooter made their intentions known. To laugh it off could cost someone their life.

11. Establish, maintain, and promote a positive working relationship with your local policing agencies.

12. Many schools in New York State are fortunate to have NYS troopers, sheriffs, and local police officers in their schools during the year. These unscheduled visits each day provide a presence of security that is emotionally positive. Would-be attackers are challenged by the nonexistence of routine and thus this is an excellent layer of school safety and security. The U.S. Department of Homeland Security suggests encouraging law enforcement personnel to have a presence in your school, such as having lunch in the cafeteria or completing administrative work in the school library, a patrol car in the school parking lot or even an empty office. Their presence can equate to deterrence, much the same as a school resource officer (SRO).

13. Ensure that your speaker system can be heard in every nook and cranny of your district. An all-call for a lockdown must lock down your buildings completely with one simple statement. Practice this, and have the students practice this. Everyone needs to know how to make this call. When the situation appears, it may not be an adult near the phone, so students (grade 8 and up) must know how to do this.

14. Do not call a lockdown for an incident in one building in your district, call for an entire district lockdown instead. The first issue may be a screen for something larger in another location.

15. SROs are promoted as the perfect step for school safety and security. Ironically, they are barely mentioned in the ASIS white paper and the documents from the Department of Homeland Security and the Secret Service. In Columbine Klebold and Harris attacked the cafeteria first as the SRO ate lunch there at the same time every day. The Red Lake School Massacre found the attacker targeting and killing the SRO at the beginning of the massacre.

    Perpetrators often know the school layout, class schedule, and the SROs habits. As such they can plan around routines in order to strike with more efficiency. This element, when an SRO does not have a routine, adds a challenging step toward deterring violence. Both Parkland and Santa Fe had SROs and both schools were victims of school shootings. SROs are an excellent layer of defense, but there are a host of other strategies that need to be equally in place.

16. Lastly, never assume you know how someone will react. Talking about school safety and security, acting out mock drills, and reading about it is quite different from the day when you will be called to implement this training. To increase the odds that people will do what is needed to protect all human life, trainings need to occur annually. Ensure that the people with the right disposition have the right job for when an event occurs. Being the superintendent does not necessarily equate with being the best person to oversee a command post. Be honest and assign positions to people who will get the job done when called upon.

Once a safety plan is developed it must be clearly articulated to the entire staff and to some degree to the students. Staff need to know what to do and when. Students also need to know what to do and how to do it. Practicing lockdown drills will aid in the development and internalization of this knowledge. Annual training is required by many states, and schools should seek to meet the minimum requirement and add more training if possible.

Many states have reduced the number of mandatory fire drills for schools and increased the number of safety drills such as lockdowns, lockouts, and evacuation drills. To maximize the internalization the process has to be implemented with integrity and fidelity. Drills should take place during lunch, in between periods, prior to the start of the school day, at the end of the school day, and after school.

After the drills it is imperative to have open meetings with students (grade and age appropriate) to answer questions and to provide a calm atmosphere where they can express their feelings and thoughts. This is also true for staff. When planning training days, it is highly recommended to equally plan time for debriefing.

Along with lockdown, lockout, and evacuation drills, the reunification drill must take place. In the event of an active shooter, no matter how the situation plays out, at the end of the event the school will need to reunite students with their parents. Emotions will be running high and rational thought will be hard to find. Therefore, like the fire drills, lockdown, lockout, and evacuation, schools must practice how they will unite families.

Practicing a reunification drill goes well with the evacuation drill. This type of drill could take place the day before a vacation thus allowing families a little head start. This would increase the odds of less push-back.

Reunification requires appropriate assignments of staff based upon personality and grit. It would be improper to assign a quiet introvert the job of standing at the door where parents will enter when called upon. Given that rational thought is out the window during this high-stress moment, the quiet introvert will be pushed aside. Think bouncer and assign someone who fits this bill.

Understand the size of your building when choosing the site for the reunification. Communication is going to be key, thus denoting the need for speakerphones. Buy these. Practice with them, and keep extra batteries in a location where the speakerphone is stored.

Students may be in the reunification site for quite some time before the arrival of their parents. As such school leaders should have plans for keeping the students calm and orderly (as best as can be expected). One elementary school in the New York State has the local movie theater as the reunification site. Students will be kept in the main theater so that siblings can be together. Theater personnel have authorized showing movies during the time the students are in the theater. They provided the key to the principal for the movie cabinet and also trained a few of the school staff on how to load the movies. A calming distraction will help de-escalate the stress of the children.

It is essential to practice all safety drills throughout the year. Staff and students need to practice the drills and be allowed time afterward to debrief. Practice drills with law enforcement as opportunity allows. Each drill, training, and debrief will provide valuable information on how to tweak and improve the plan.

In today's day and age, it goes without saying that everyone is on the same page when it comes to preventing aggression in schools. Prevention is possible. There are resources available to school leaders through law enforcement as well as third-party vendors to assist in prevention strategies. TAP App Security and CLPS Consultancy Group are two such third-party vendors that offer a digital format for crisis management in schools. Along with third-party options the U.S. Secret Service and the FBI equally offer procedures for enacting a threat assessment process to ensure a proactive measure is in place. Additionally, the ASIS white paper (2016) is available to the public and it also offers insight into a proactive process. Numerous sources with the same message create the process and ensure that everyone in the organization is aware of how it functions.

To be proactive in a school setting requires what is commonly known as situational awareness. This simple concept is taught in driver education courses as it seeks to ensure that the driver looks not only at the road but also at the factors that may affect their travel on the road. School safety requires situational awareness for the same reason.

"Cooper's Color Codes" were designed by a Jeff Cooper for use in tactical training (ASIS, 2016, p. 11). Cooper's Color Codes (see table 3.1) apply color to the varying levels of situation awareness.

Operating at the *yellow level is optimum* for school leaders. This can only occur when there are open lines of communication with faculty, staff, and students. There may be a false sense of safety if incident reports regarding bullying, disrespect, or inappropriate comments are not making their way to school leaders. This may be occurring due to a serious issue, and that may be that students have lost faith in the system. Should students or staff feel that nothing will happen if they report an issue or incident, a dangerous path may ensue. It is human nature for people to choose to take action on their own when they feel as though no one else will do so. The most dangerous person is the one who feels as though they have nothing to lose.

To assist in creating an environment where the faculty, staff, and students feel safe and comfortable reporting issues or concerns to school leaders, school leaders need to provide both a safe venue for reporting as well as an established plan of action for assessing all reports. First and foremost, there should be an anonymous platform for reporting. One option to address this is to have a portal on the school web page where reports can be entered. There are third-party vendors who assist in the "see or hear something, say something" reporting and can create options for schools. Anonymous reporting options are critical.

Many people consider the attack at Columbine High School to be the catalyst for future copycat endeavors. The Columbine, Colorado, community continues to deal with this atrocity as people travel there every year to look at

Table 3.1   Cooper's Color Codes Indicate Levels of Situational Awareness

Cooper's Color Codes	
WHITE	Unprepared and unready to take action
YELLOW	Prepared, alert, and relaxed. Good situational awareness.
ORANGE	Alert to probable danger. Ready to take action.
RED	Action mode. Focused on the emergency at hand.
BLACK	Panic. Breakdown of physical and mental performance.

Source: ASIS International School Safety & Security Council (2016).

the place where the horrific attack occurred. Unlike Sandy Hook Elementary School, Columbine High School remains an operational school building. To prevent the constant deluge of strangers stopping by to view the school, the Sandy Hook school was demolished with a new elementary school built on the same property but not on the footprint of the original building.

KEY IDEAS TO REMEMBER

First responders will arrive with sirens blaring and lights flashing. They will go through hell and high water to get to the school in distress. If nothing else, this chapter informs school leaders on how to buy time from the moment the incident is announced to the arrival of law enforcement.

To begin the process of determining what needs to be done in your school district, and in each building, the STAT must complete an overall audit to determine the baseline for all buildings. Many of these actions cost nothing more than time and an adjustment to a new normal, such as keeping all classroom doors closed and locked at all times, conducting annual safety drills, making sure active shooter drills occur in each of the district's buildings, ensuring lines of open and honest communication with staff and students, and practicing reunification drills.

The initial active shooter event will be over in less than 10 minutes, but the reunification process will take much more time. Be cognizant of where you are choosing to set your reunification site for each building. It may make sense at first to put the district together, but this would be a mistake as it will intensify an already stressful event. Be sure to put the right people in the appropriate roles for this juncture. Seniority is out the window in determining who should do what. What matters for this crucial time, when emotions and anxiety are high, is a setting where the school leaders and staff can help reunite parents and children in a calm and efficient manner. This takes precise planning and practice.

School resource officers have been in existence for decades and are now in the limelight as a hopeful deterrent to active shooters. The reality is that all written documents concerning safety and security refer to the actions threat assessment teams can take for their schools. This includes having a safety vestibule in the entryway of each school building, ensuring the right person is manning this position, and overseeing the implementation of safety measures in each building. School resource officers fall further down on the list of possible deterrents.

This is not to say that their position and presence is not beneficial. That is hardly the case, as SROs do more than just police the buildings. They become an advocate for students, a mentor, and a source of information for both students and staff. A sense of peace takes hold of the school community when a uniformed law enforcement officer is in the building.

For district's that are unable to afford an SRO there are other steps that can be taken. Development of a good working relationship with all law enforcement agencies that work within the district is optimal. Offer them a space in the district to work on paperwork and make phone calls. It is their presence and that of the squad car out front that makes an impression on would-be attackers. Request all active agencies in the district that they conduct walkthroughs of the school buildings during the day. This allows them an opportunity to really get to know the buildings, students, and staff. And lastly, offering free coffee or water for them when they stop by is not a bad option. Anything that entices their presence is worth its weight in gold.

Finally, it is imperative that school leaders now function under code yellow, from Cooper's Color Codes. Prepared, alert, and relaxed goes a long way in optimizing situational awareness for the district. When something appears to be out of the norm it is important to investigate it and if need be hand it over to the DRA. Situational awareness should be practiced in numerous aspects of our lives, including a trip to the grocery store, mall, movie theater, and so on. The United States has borne witness to a multitude of school shootings this past decade, and as such it is important that we, as citizens, do our part to protect ourselves and our families. Being cognizant of our situational awareness will go far in protecting all that we love.

Chapter 4

Threat Assessment in Action

At first I was one of those who complained about these ridiculous drills that take time away from instruction. After today's drill, and yeah, just a drill, I have changed my mind. We need to do this every year and for each building.

A new normal is occurring across the nation as school districts, community leaders, legislators, law enforcement, state education departments, and federal agencies work to instill safety and security measures without making schools cold, hard institutions. This is an incredibly important balancing act, as schools at their very core need to be seen and felt as embodying a nurturing learning environment. Therefore, the challenge is to install safety and security measures without negatively impacting the serenity and supportive atmosphere of a school.

The deadly shooting at Columbine occurred twenty years ago, and this tragedy has become the reference point in regard to active shooters. This tragedy claimed the lives of 13 people and in turn has become somewhat of a tourist issue. Over the years the intrigue with the school has dwindled a bit, but people still try to peer into the windows, ask for tours, and a few copycat individuals were apprehended by law enforcement.

The high school buildings and campus of Columbine still stand amid a bit of controversy as some would like the building torn down and rebuilt. In Newtown, Connecticut, voters approved the demolition of the Sandy Hook Elementary School. The rebuilt school is a distance from the former building and today houses state-of-the-art safety measures that schools across the country are seeking to mimic. Marjory Stoneman Douglas High School in Parkland, Florida, is also contemplating demolishing the building in an effort to remove the constant reminder of the deadly shooting from 2018.

In regard to practical advice, it is important to remember the past in order to prevent its repetition in the present. By removing the school buildings where the atrocities occurred, the school districts are able to limit the idolization of the event to a certain degree. In their places, new schools with current safety and security features will be installed and all staff properly trained on school safety and security.

Following the murders at Parkland High School, the state of Florida created a commission to study what happened with a lens on how to prevent such an atrocity in the future. The commission included members of law enforcement, educational leaders, attorneys, and 2 parents of children who died that fateful day. The final report is over 400 pages of analysis and includes areas where the school district fell short of providing a safe and secure learning environment.

When the new Sandy Hook Elementary School was constructed law enforcement members were invited to tour the facility that housed state-of-the-art safety and security elements. From these tours law enforcement personnel were able to bring back to the school districts in their communities' ideas for improving safety and security. Some ideas come with hefty price tags, and yet others required merely changing the current state of operations within the schools that only cost time.

Given the time frame needed for first responders to arrive, the following advice is offered from the SSSC white paper, documents provided by the U.S. Departments of Homeland Security and the Secret Service, recommendations from NYS troopers, numerous articles, and papers from security professionals and legal advice following the Parkland shootings. First, it is imperative to understand that your school/school district will become a victim of an aggressor. The only unknown is when and where.

1. Continue safety drills and discussions with both students and staff. The last fire in a school that claimed a victim was in the 1950s and the last school shooting was at the close of this past year. Students need to feel empowered to come forward without any fear of reprisal or disbelief. A warm and caring school culture goes a long way in establishing this empowerment.

   Some people argue that practicing active shooter drills is traumatic for both staff and students, and that this practice should not occur. There is some merit to this argument in that the drills are not stand-alone events; rather, there needs to be communication with the school leaders and the school community. Prior to the drills the following topics should be discussed with all stakeholders: Why are we conducting this drill; how will it play out; what is my role/responsibility; what is the role of the first responders; who are the first responders; and how fast will they get here?

It would be extremely beneficial to also have representation from local law enforcement at some of these discussions.

2. Conduct social-emotional discussions with students as part of a threat assessment team approach. Give the people on the team the purview and authority to act. Prevention is the optimal goal.
3. Harden the school to prevent it from becoming a target. Are your classroom doors easily breached; do you have a safety vestibule in each building; where are the panic buttons; can every classroom phone announce a lockdown and dial out to access 911? The intruder will get into your building; the question is how you can best protect the children and the staff until the first responders arrive. Bullet-resistant glass and solid core doors that are kept locked at all times will help to buy valuable time.

   A factor that affected many school shootings is the fact that staff were unable to lock the doors from the inside. The failure to be able to conduct this simple task resulted in the deaths of students and staff.
4. Key people need to attend threat assessment and school safety trainings together. The discussions held afterward and common language will go a long way in helping to prepare and protect the school community. The U.S. Secret Service Department advocates that a threat assessment process is an effective facet for school safety.

   Use clear language. "Red Alert" may sound important but a clear "Lockdown" leaves no scope for alternative interpretations.

   School safety trainings need to include the active shooter training, lockdowns, lockouts, as well as sheltering drills. Additionally, students need to be involved in the training and they additionally need time to talk about this with school leaders and/or their teachers. Students will have questions and concerns and their voice needs to be heard. A two-way conversation needs to be established. Processes for reporting concerns, anonymously, must be expressly presented to students (as appropriate by age and cognitive ability).
5. Active shooter training needs to occur in each building in your district. After such a training was completed at an elementary school, one of the teachers stated the need to do this in each building due to the difference in layouts and personnel.
6. Be sure to plan time for teachers and staff to ask questions. Presenting and training is a large part of the security equation, but time has to be devoted to ensure internalization. In the classroom it is referred to as checking for understanding and closure. Practice what is preached to our staff.
7. Single point of entry for each building, no exceptions. Be sure to have protocols for how the single point of entry will be operated. Decide who will man the door, what process will be in place to determine who may or

may not enter the building, and what needs to occur when someone who is not allowed entry becomes aggravated and aggressive.

Most school districts have implemented the single point of entry process over a decade ago. However, most plans are fully functional only during the school day. Plans and protocols need to be in place after school when play practice, sports practice and games, and extra help are taking place. It is highly irregular for schools to be emptied once the final bell rings. Rather, schools are very active with extracurricular and community events after the last bell rings. Districts must provide security when the school buildings are in use. It is a societal expectation that when children are within the confines of the school that they will be safe.

8. Make sure that school buildings have well-lit exteriors and cameras are able to view every angle of the buildings both internally and externally. Lighting and visibility are critical aspects to have in place to help prevent incidents and to help ascertain what is happening during an incident.
9. Students should never be allowed to use a teacher's key/swipe card—ever!
10. All visitors must sign in/sign out and use school designated IDs that are single use. Never have a set visitor tag that can be used throughout the year. Instead the tag should be printed each day, and clearly display the date of the approved visitation.
11. Visitors should not be allowed to bring bags into schools. A no-bag policy takes some time to get used to, but so did removing our shoes at airports.
12. People working the front desks (where visitors are allowed in) should be staffed by those who know the students and community well. Never staff this position with a substitute.
13. All staff must wear their ID at work at all times.
14. Enforce a zero-tolerance policy regarding joking about school shootings and mass killings. This supports the federal statute that makes even a joke of a terrorist threat punishable with minimum of 3 years in prison.
15. Establish, maintain, and promote a positive working relationship with your local policing agencies.

Some NYS schools are fortunate to have NYS troopers, sheriffs, and local police officers in their schools daily throughout the year. These unscheduled visits provide a presence of security that is emotionally positive. Would-be attackers are challenged by the nonexistence of routine and thus this is an excellent layer of school safety and security.

The following is recommended by the U.S. Department of Homeland Security: "Where school resource officers are not present, encourage law enforcement personnel to have a presence in your school, such as having lunch in the cafeteria or completing administrative work in the school library, a patrol car in the school parking lot or even an empty office." Presence can equate to deterrence.

16. Ensure that your speaker system can be heard in every nook and cranny of your district. An all-call for a lockdown must lock down your buildings completely.

17. When you call a lockdown for an incident in one building in your district, call for an entire district lockdown instead. If there is an issue in one building within the district, it is imperative to lock down the entire district as the initial issue could be a diversionary tactic.

18. All schools need to have adequate surveillance videos. High-definition cameras now allow for real-time imaging that will allow law enforcement and first responders vital information.

    In Parkland the camera/surveillance system was on a delay. First responders were not informed of this crucial fact. In fact the system was delayed by several minutes. When law enforcement first responders moved to apprehend the shooter, he was no longer there.

19. School resource officers are promoted as the perfect step for school safety and security. Ironically, they are barely mentioned in the SSSC white paper and the documents from the Department of Homeland Security and the Secret Service.

    In Columbine, Klebold and Harris attacked the cafeteria first as the SRO ate lunch there at the same time every day. The Red Lake School Massacre found the attacker targeting and killing the SRO at the beginning of the massacre. According to an excerpt in the SSSC white paper: "Often, the perpetrators of K-12 violence are known—either current students or former students, staff or teachers" (SSSC, 2016, p.39). They know the school layout, class schedule, and have become familiarized with the SROs habits. They know when and where to strike with least resistance and most effect. Deterring school violence under these circumstances is very difficult."

Both Parkland and Santa Fe had SROs and both schools were the victims of school shootings. School resource officers are an excellent layer of defense, but a host of other strategies need to be equally in place.

These 19 points of practical advice include areas that are simple to implement and others that will require lengthy discussions and planning in order to begin implementation. School leaders are taxed with numerous expectations from the federal, state, and local community in terms of academic performance and fiduciary responsibilities. The added layer of school safety and security is critical but is also an additional layer of expectations.

Some of the school safety and security advice offered above comes at no cost to the district. Rather, the only cost is the time it takes to create a new normal in regard to protocols and procedures. Single point of entry took a little getting used to, but no one questions this procedure any more. Implementing the same procedures after school may renew the grumbling. Just as TSA wait lines at airports have caused initial angst, it is no longer argued about. Having to spend a little more time prior to arriving at the gate is now expected and accepted. Knowing that the reason for this is to improve safety and security helped to enable its implementation with relatively few issues. The same is true for schools.

School leaders should not try to develop and implement safety and security procedures in isolation. These plans need to include stakeholders who will help to spread the message of the new normal. Establish a district-wide committee that is comprised of the superintendent, director of buildings and grounds, building principals, union presidents, representation from local law enforcement, and if possible a parent, a board member, and a community mental health professional. These need to be district-level decisions and not left to individual buildings. The plans will affect all students and staff, and as such, there cannot be differing terms or procedures.

Once the team is developed it then becomes an act of prioritization. Start with what can be implemented immediately and at little to no cost. Draft the language so that it is clear and easily understood. Create an ad-hoc committee from the safety and security team that will be charged with communicating the language so that all staff and students can clearly understand what is expected.

The larger items that require funding then become a task for the superintendent and board member as they need to incorporate these into the budget development process. School communities have been very supportive of school safety endeavors that have been incorporated into budgets.

Lastly, it is important for school leaders to have open lines of communication with local law enforcement and first responders. Keep abreast of all information published on the topic of school safety from the U.S. Secret Service, U.S. Department of Homeland Security, the U.S. Department of Defense, and of course the state Department of Education. If nothing else, they will inform everyone on any latest developments that may be cause for concern or implementation. This is an ongoing issue, and unfortunately there is no end date to update safety and security plans and implementation.

KEY IDEAS TO REMEMBER

This chapter focused on implementing a threat assessment plan along with 19 points of practical advice. It is imperative to understand, acknowledge, and internalize the realization that schools have to operate under a new normal. This new normal blends safety and security measures with a nurturing learning environment. A balance can be achieved so that students and staff are safe and secure in an environment that is hardened but not to the point where it is akin to a prison, quite the epitome of a balancing act.

History finds school shootings beginning as early as 1840, although the more common reference point is Columbine which occurred in 1999. A plethora of copycat shootings have occurred since then and with each violent attack America renews the pledge to stop this from happening again. This chapter accepts that challenge and offers practical advice for implementing a threat assessment for schools.

The fact is that there will be another active shooter attempt with the only unknown being when and where. The question then stands out, "Are you prepared and ready for such an attempt?" Nineteen points are offered to help school leaders prepare and prevent aggressive attacks on schools through threat assessment pedagogy. Many of these strategies cost nothing but time and energy to implement. How well they function is based upon the adoption of a new normal in regard to operational procedures for both students and staff.

A single point of entry is effective only when it is used as the only point of entry. Whether school is in session or not, whether it is cold and rainy or hot and muggy, the only entry into the building must be the single point of entry. This entry will always be staffed by someone who knows the community well and is vigilant about not letting anyone in who does not have legitimate business to conduct inside the school walls. The security vestibule is a critical factor in ensuring that the single point of entry is effective. Whereas the delivery person or parent dropping off soccer cleats may gain access to the entryway, they do not have a valid reason to enter into the main building. A majority of school shooters have entered through the front door. They are brazen and determined, so cutting off this access point is an effective tool.

Solid core doors with bullet-resistant glass are only an effective security and safety tool when the doors are left closed and locked all day. This may be an inconvenience at first, but so were the TSA agents at the airport when they first arrived. A little inconvenience for safety is something we can all live with.

Finally, if not already in place, school districts need to create threat assessment teams. This group must include school administrators and representatives of the district, including, but not limited to, the school nurse, director of buildings and grounds, and teachers. Once established this team needs to establish a quarterly meeting schedule (at the very least) and begin work by determining the security baseline for the school: what is in place, what is needed, what needs updating, and so on. Prioritize the list with what can be done immediately due to no cost, and then prepare your plan for the rest. Communicate this plan with the board of education and the full staff. Implementation of cost-free strategies needs to be in place immediately. Train your staff and students, run the drills, and debrief often with all stakeholders. Research, plan, implement, review, repeat, repeat, repeat.

Chapter 5

Dangerousness Risk Assessment Protocols

Assessment teams and protocols allow for the ability to identify and prevent acts of violence from escalating. Attackers do not snap; they simply put their plan into action.

As described in detail in chapter 3, the school threat assessment plan is a set plan that is reviewed and updated at least annually. It is activated when an individual(s) or the school is facing a threat to their safety. The school threat assessment plan will require ongoing reassessment of the current evolving threat to guide the decision-making process as the situation unfolds. The plan must contain the names and contact information of the people on the School Threat Assessment Team (STAT) and their assigned responsibilities. It typically involves a multidisciplinary approach that includes people with intimate knowledge of the site and its inhabitants, multiple law enforcement agencies, emergency services, tactical emergency services, mental health personnel trained in threat assessment, the school psychologist, and so on. The incident commander will be the administrator named in the plan, at least until a senior law enforcement official arrives on scene, at which time the officer will assume operational jurisdiction.

The threat assessment plan is implemented as written and approved when an incident or potential threat is acknowledged. However, it is understood that every situation will have unique variables that require individual finesse. The plan must be implemented as close as possible as it was crafted with clear heads and input from experts. That being said, Helmuth von Moltke the Elder, who was the chief of staff of the Prussian Army once stated: "No battle plan survives first contact with the enemy." This quote is relevant to the issue at hand, as it takes into account the numerous variables an active threat presents to a school district or community. The school threat assessment plan is utilized for assessing and reassessing the current potential threat. It will be revised and updated as data is gathered about the unfolding threat.

For example, if the district's physical plant changes due to a boiler failure requiring a replacement boiler that only fits in another location, then the school threat assessment plan will need to be reviewed and updated again. If the wrestling coach assigned the task of manning the ingress and egress of family members at the reunification site moved to another county, the school threat assessment plan will need to be updated with his replacement, who must become intimately familiar with the entire plan. The devil is in the details.

When the situation is considered an active threat, the school threat assessment plan is the boilerplate for all activities moving forward. It may need to evolve and expand as circumstances dictate. The incident commander will make any decisions that vary from the written plan. This allows for incorporating new information and necessary strategic plan updates to maintain a secure and safe environment.

As the STAT is investigating the potential threat and gathering data, their analysis may find a need to conduct a DRA. This generally occurs when the STAT find grievances, resentments, or changes in behavior, and cannot ascertain if the person(s) of interest has the ability to act upon their angst. As the STAT finds increased warning signs, the DRA becomes the prominent focus (see figure 5.1). The DRA team is a subset of the STAT team, and as such will have intimate knowledge of the situation with the authorization to take action as needed. Consider them the safety SWAT team for the school.

At this point, the school threat assessment is being conducted by the STAT and they are continuously evaluating the evolving situation. This is a multidisciplinary team that includes people that know the site and its inhabitants, multiple law enforcement agencies, emergency services and tactical emergency services, mental health personnel trained in threat assessment, and so on, all of who train and work off the threat assessment plan. If the threat spreads to multiple noncontiguous or even contiguous sites, then subsidiary

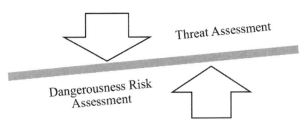

Figure 5.1 As the STAT Finds Increased Warning Signs the DRA Becomes the Prominent Focus. *Source*: Self-Designed.

STAT and threat assessment plans may become necessary for each site. Think of it as one large battlefield splitting into two battlefields, each with its site specific strategic plan changes and STAT.

The chart below shows a pictorial representation of threat assessment, overall STAT, and STAT1 and STAT2 for two separate sites of concern. An example of this would be two shooters at different sites, even if their sites are contiguous with one another. All of the data flows to the individual command center from each of the threat assessment sites.

The part of threat assessment that looks specifically at the Person of Interest (POI) identified as possibly linked to the threat is called dangerousness risk assessment, or DRA. There can potentially be more than one possible threatening person, in which case each suspect will need to have their own DRA: DRA1 and DRA2. The DRA teams are subsets of the STATs and should include the school administrators, psychologist, counselor, at least one teacher, and the multidisciplinary team described above, such as multiple law enforcement agencies, emergency services and tactical emergency services, mental health personnel trained in threat assessment, and so on (figure 5.2).

This kind of organizational construct will allow for detailed documentation to be attached to appropriate locations and suspects. As a standard flow chart, it can expand to cover as many sites and suspects as are potentially involved. All of the subsidiary STATs and DRAs will keep school theater command's threat assessment team informed. If strategies must change, theater command

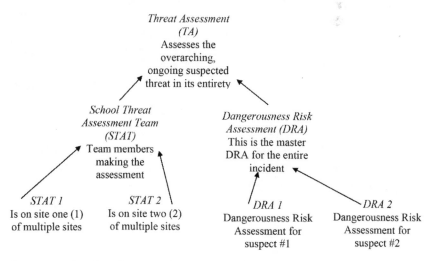

Figure 5.2   Flowchart for How Threat Assessment and DRA Work in Tandem. *Source:* Self-Designed.

will communicate that to STATs and DRA teams. It's like the music has changed keys, yet everyone still plays in unison.

Sadly, violence in America's schools has become too common. People are impacted in large numbers, just because someone holds a resentment of one kind or another that could be easily resolved with simple conversation. And yet they are not. What if we could identify those at increased risk of behaving dangerously, either toward themselves or toward others, and successfully intervene before they act?

Can we predict violent events? Unfortunately no! There is no person or test that can accurately predict or even postdict a violent act. We cannot look forward in time and say who will commit a violent act and when. In fact, we cannot go back in time to a known violent event, complete a forensic psychiatric autopsy, and determine how we could have predicted those past acts of violence. Even highly trained and experienced mental health professionals and law enforcement personnel are no better at predicting future violent acts than the flip of a coin. Even people planning to commit their egregious acts cannot accurately predict them, because they can suddenly change their plans or their minds at any time.

Does this mean the situation is hopeless? Absolutely not! We can become extremely good at recognizing *indicators* that a person is at increased risk of behaving dangerously, so that an intervention can be made before they act that will mitigate or even eliminate their risk of committing a violent act.

Mass shooters in schools have consistently been very open and accurate about proclaiming their intentions to commit their horrific acts. They have done this primarily through texting and social media. In some instances they also spoke to other people directly about their violent intentions and/or recorded their intentions on their mobile device and then sent it to various people. Others made flyers and posters that were hung at various locations around the school building.

Eric Harris and Dylan Klebold did not just wake up on April 20, 1999, and decide at that point to attack the students and staff at Columbine High School. Rather, they began incubating their mass murder attack approximately three years earlier when they started posting violent statements on an online gaming site. Their violent comments were reported and this is the sad part, as that is where the investigation began and ended. Working as a Monday morning quarterback it is evident that after that day many other warning signs were simply missed or not addressed.

For two relatively normal kids, their behavior escalated to the point where they were subsequently arrested for stealing, increased their fascination with weapons and bomb-making, made and posted a "Hit Men for Hire" video, amassed weapons and ammunition, and finally built explosive devices in their parent's garage. At 11:19 a.m. they began the mass murder of peers and staff and at 12:08 p.m. they committed suicide. Forty-eight minutes of pure terror. The only real warning was a message to a friend at 11:18 a.m. to go home. Unfortunately, at the time of this mass killing there was no such thing as a STAT.

If a DRA team had existed in Columbine in 1996, it is highly likely that the change in Dylan Klebold and Eric Harris's behaviors and personalities would have triggered a thorough investigation. Their video, homemade bombs, and an arsenal of weapons and ammunition would have been found prior to their use. Pre-attack indicators (PAINs) were evident. According to the "Active Shooter" white paper (SSSC, 2016), it is imperative that observations of subtle PAINs be investigated as it is quite rare to actually find a direct threat preceding an attack.

Do not wait until there is an actual threat of danger as it will be too late at that point and operations will be at the Cooper's Color Code Black level where panic and breakdown of physical and mental performance occurs. PAINs actions that may flag the need to further investigate include, but are not limited to,

- threat of suicide or self-harm;
- threat of violence (directly or implied);
- fascination with/asserting ownership of firearms;
- history of violence; behavior obviously insensitive to others;
- preoccupation with themes of violence;
- intimidating others; frequently confrontational;
- crossing boundaries (excessive calls, emails, etc.);
- marked academic performance decline;
- notable changes in personality, mood, or behavior;
- giving away personal possessions;
- noticeable decline in personal hygiene; and
- substance abuse.

SSSC white paper, 2016

When developing a DRA team the natural team leader is the building administrator. In this role the principal has full authority to take action and this is critical for a successful assessment team. All members of the team need to have authority to act. Any bureaucracy that requires additional approval only muddies the water and delays action.

DRA teams allow school districts the ability to identify and prevent acts of violence. These teams have three main functions, which are identify, assess, and manage the threat. Once the threat is made known, the DRA team will meet to begin the process of collecting data. Data will come from school data, family data as well as outside data. School data will come from discussions with teachers, teaching assistants, bus drivers, cafeteria staff, and other personnel. Discussions may take place in person or electronically. Family data discussions will take place with parents/guardians, siblings, and any other relatives who may have firsthand knowledge. Outside data may be available from neighbors, friends, employers, or coaches, and so on.

The discussions for each data set will seek to find the answers to the same set of direct questions. Questions for consideration when conducting a DRA are included in figure 5.3.

The questions address two main areas of concern: bullying and access to weapons. Bullying, or the perception of being bullied, is considered to be a serious risk factor for schools. Chronic/ongoing bullying may lead to depression and other neuropsychological problems in a student. If left unaddressed, or perceived to be unaddressed, the student may feel as though they have nothing to lose. Mental distress tends to develop which further escalates the issue.

Access to weapons is a critical factor when assessing a person's penchant for violence. Remember, the greater the frequency, intensity, and especially the variety of violence and/or weapons the attacker has been exposed to, the greater their risk for acting violently now. Venting about or toying with the idea of attacking people or property is quite different from doing those things while having access to the tools and means for carrying it out. *Access*

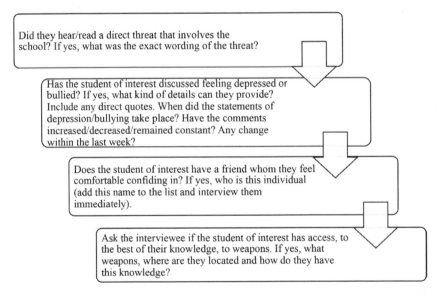

Figure 5.3 Questions for Consideration When Conducting a DRA. *Source:* Self-Designed, MS Word.

to weapons and the ability to cause harm is the tipping point that makes this a credible threat. Ability to act upon the plan to attack and/or cause harm is readily available and all that remains is the decision to act. *Attackers do not snap; they simply put their plan into action.*

It is imperative that interviews be conducted in a calm and professional manner. At this point the team members are operating at Cooper's Orange and Red levels of situational awareness resulting in a strong flow of adrenaline. In order for the interviewees to feel comfortable in discussing the POI, the interviewer must check their personal feelings.

Secondly, throughout the interview the interviewer must remain focused on the questions and the answers being provided. In doing so they must ensure that the questions are understood, and that the answers actually convey what the interviewee intended. In order to do this it is suggested that the interviewer ask the interviewee if they understand each question before the answer is provided. Once the question is answered the reply should be paraphrased back to the interviewee or if possible restated verbatim. Direct quotes from the interviewee are extremely helpful.

It is important that the interview occur in a room with little distractions and in a manner that presents the interviewer as nonjudgmental. If the interviewee is open to the concept of recording the interview, this is an optimal strategy to ensure proper recording of the meeting. Include at the very start of the recording a direct question to the interviewee asking for their permission to record the interview. With this state the date and start time of the interview and then end the recording by once again stating the date and end time of the interview.

Digital software is available through third parties for organizing the interviews for threat assessment teams and DRA teams. Both the threat assessment and DRA teams must ensure proper maintenance of all data related to discipline, especially threats to a school, students or staff. This type of data must be separate from student management systems according to rules and guidance from the Family Educational Rights and Privacy Act (FERPA), state and national standards guidelines. To prevent students of concern from falling through the cracks there needs to be a set program for maintaining critical information regarding threats. Sturdy, bound, professional style journals work well and don't require someone to sit with their face glued to a screen or monitor, thereby losing sight of the very person they should be interested in getting to know. Most people can handwrite well enough without looking at the paper. All documentation must be maintained in a secured area that is accessible by the school leaders, and DRA team. The FERPA must be maintained.

Once the data has been completed the team must reconvene with all data available for review. The DRA team will be led by the building administrator and should also include a variety of disciplines. Teams should include, but not be limited to, teachers, guidance counselors, coaches, mental health professionals, administrators, and school resource officers should the district employ them (NTAC, 2000, p. 3).

According to the Secret Service Operational Guide for Preventing School Violence (2000) the assessment team must have prescribed protocols and procedures. The team needs to practice these procedures throughout the year and not wait until a threat occurs to run through the process. Protocol is required for identifying who will interview the student(s) of interest, as well as all the ancillary people such as classmates, teachers, parents, guardians, and neighbors.

Additionally, these interviews need to be documented and maintained in a format that is readily accessible to all DRA team members. Teams must meet on a regular basis and review the plan often so that when an issue happens they are ready to act without hesitation.

The threshold for what incidents/issues trigger an assessment team review should be set very low. It is better to review an issue to end up determining it is not a credible threat than to pass on an issue that appears to be minor only to end up dealing with a full-blown attack on the school or a student. At the very least, the interviews will allow for a thorough review of the acting culture which may in the long run result in changing of school policies or procedures. Knowledge is powerful.

The team should develop a set threshold for when law enforcement will be brought in. This should be set in concrete and not open for interpretation. Facts need to precede emotion when establishing these hard lines for when to bring in law enforcement. At this level law enforcement will equally conduct a threat assessment and very well may determine it to be non-credible. It is far safer to pass it up the line to get confirmation than to make a judgment call that may not be in the best interest of the school community.

The NTAC advises that when reviewing threat assessment data teams need to look for emerging themes as they relate to the student's actions and overall circumstances. In doing so where the threat may not be deemed credible, the team may be able to discern actions to be taken to prevent this student from further escalating their behavior. It is critical that the team look for stressors in the child's life to help explain the path that they are embarking on. This includes looking holistically at the child's life, both in and out of school. Providing timely interventions such as guidance, mentoring, or mental health therapy may help de-escalate and save a child in crisis.

Once the data is reviewed the team then chooses whether the threat is credible or not. If the threat is not deemed credible, all the documentation needs to be saved. When the threat is deemed credible the team then must decide if it is something that the school can address or a call must be made to law enforcement for legal action. Once law enforcement is involved and they deem the threat to be credible they will assume control of the situation.

Evidence collected during the threat assessment will aid law enforcement as they implement their protocols.

KEY IDEAS TO REMEMBER

In this chapter, DRA was introduced. Dangerous risk assessment teams focus on gathering as much information as possible about the suspected actors, which can be used to mitigate or even eliminate the threat(s), hopefully without any untoward incidents. Although there does not exist an ability to predict or postdict with accuracy a violent act, it is possible to recognize indicators that an individual is at increased risk for behaving dangerously.

A threat assessment team focuses on the entire threat landscape, including the threat campus or campuses, preparations to prevent a threat from proceeding to becoming an act, and what to do when a threat is determined to be possible or real. Taking a Monday morning quarterback approach to active shooter incidents since 1840 one commonality stands out: the active shooters, whether directly or indirectly, made their intentions known.

The optimal point for intervention in hopes of mitigating or preventing the violent act from happening is when the actor(s) begin expressing their grievances and resentments. This may occur through verbal or written statements. Additionally, there are also PAINS to be aware of. These 12 indicators were developed post Columbine and focus on a change in a person's demeanor.

Of particular interest in regard to the PAINs indicators is the perception of being bullied. Whether real or not, just the perception caused them to manifest this issue as a grievance and then resentment. Add in accessibility to weapons and the DRA team now has a credible threat that will warrant calling in law enforcement (if not already on the team).

Dangerous risk assessment teams are a subset of the STAT. It is critical to follow author Jim Collins's advice on this and have the right people on the bus. Seniority goes out the window with this team. Cool, focused, and level-headed individuals, who are charged with the power to act, need to be on this team. They will have specific protocols and procedures that include how data will be shared, how to conduct the interviews, what questions will be asked, who will be interviewed and by whom, and lastly it will be clear how and where all this information will be maintained.

When conducting a DRA, the team members will look for emerging themes. Once a determination is made, the team will decide whether to handle the issue internally or hand it off to law enforcement. The tipping point for this decision generally, but not always, focuses on accessibility to weapons. If a possible attacker has weapons, or access to weapons, law enforcement must take over the case.

Chapter 6

Dangerousness Risk Assessment

The key is to prevent at-risk individuals from escalating on the path to violence.

Communication is the key to success. The same holds true when speaking about safety and security in our daily lives. The days of blissful innocence are no longer an option that we can engage in. Jean-Jacques Rousseau believed that man is born good and that society turns us into less civilized souls. Many people today fall into this belief that people are all good and civic minded, and do not tend to see the "bad" or "evil" in others. This is the paradigm in which humans function, and this same paradigm is often the cause of oversight or dismissiveness when someone acts or behaves out of the norm. It is time for this paradigm to change.

Sadly, violence in America's schools is becoming too common. Young people are dying in large numbers as well as getting scarred physically and/or emotionally for life. The causal denominator for this is simply that someone holds grievances and resentments that were never resolved. The answer is simple: a calm and focused conversation is needed to help the person address their real or perceived grievance and resentment. And without the conversation they behave dangerously by acting upon these grievances and resentments. There are processes that can be used every day to make the sound judgments necessary to keep society safe. The primary goal is to advance from 20/20 hindsight and Monday morning quarterbacking into the realm of 20/20 foresight with DRA.

Anyone can perform a DRA at any time just by observing and listening to the POI. Dangerousness risk assessment is defined as the critical judgment of an individual's propensity to commit a dangerous act, based upon evaluating them within the context of their social groups' policies and against a known set of risk factors. Unfortunately, there is no person or test that can accurately predict or even postdict a violent act. It is critical to fully appreciate this fact. No one can look forward in time and accurately predict who will commit a violent act and when. No one can even go back in time to a known violent event, complete a forensic psychiatric autopsy of the case, and determine how that past violent act could have been predicted. Even highly trained and experienced mental health and law enforcement professionals are no better at predicting future violent acts than the flip of a coin. In fact, even the person planning to commit the egregious act of violence cannot accurately predict it, because circumstances can suddenly change, forcing them to abandon their Plan A and deploy Plan B or create a new Plan C.

Does that mean the situation is hopeless? Absolutely not! Anyone can become extremely good at recognizing indicators that a person's risk of behaving dangerously is increasing, so that interventions can be made before they act, which will mitigate or even eliminate their risk of committing a dangerous act. This process known as DRA works for all kinds of dangerousness, including externalized violence, suicide, and even risk of accidents.

DRA will be your and your team's assessment of an individual's propensity to commit a dangerous act. Webster's Dictionary defines propensity as "an often intense natural inclination or preference." In forensic psychiatry, propensity is further delineated as being comprised of four distinct elements: frequency, imminence, likelihood, and magnitude. These elements are easily remembered using the acronym FILM. Each of the four elements should be assessed both retrospectively and prospectively, as described in table 6.1.

When **FILM**ing propensity, one must keep in the forefront of their mind these three critically important DRA facts:

1. Adolescents and young adults very openly and accurately *indicate* (not predict) their future violent plans. Therefore, do not under any circumstances ignore descriptions of where, when, or how conveyed in text messages, social media posts, emails, selfie videos, hard copy postings, and so on.
2. The greater the number, the greater the frequency, and especially the greater the variety of past violent events they have committed and/or have been exposed to, the higher their propensity to behave violently now.
3. The greater the number, the greater the frequency, and especially the greater the variety of past exposure to weapons of all kinds, the greater their propensity to behave violently now.

The definition of DRA can now be expanded upon as follows: DRA is an assessment of the often intense natural inclination or preference of an

Table 6.1   Four Elements Used by the DRA Team to Determine the Propensity for Violence

✓	Element	Description
✓	Frequency	Retrospectively, one should attempt to determine how often the person of interest (POI) has threatened with violent acts in the past, and how often those threats have been followed by an actual violent act.
		Prospectively, one wants to know how often the POI is threatening to act violently in the future.
✓	Imminence	Retrospectively, one should try to discover how soon after threatening with a violent act the POI carried it out, if at all.
		Prospectively, one wants to know how soon the violence would occur, and whether there would be any indicator that that time is approaching or is near.
✓	Likelihood	Retrospectively, one wants to determine what types of violence was the POI able to commit in the past and just how simple or complex those violent actions were.
		Prospectively, an assessment needs to be made of the likelihood that the present threat can be executed. For example, does the POI have the knowledge and/or the skill to make a pipe bomb? Does the POI have experience in using an automatic assault rifle? Does he/she have access to the means they propose to use? Does the POI have a proven history of lying or deceiving to gain attention or any other ulterior motive?
✓	Magnitude	Retrospectively, one wants to know how substantial the POI's past violent acts have been. Have they been escalating in magnitude, or have they been diminishing?
		Prospectively, an assessment needs to be made of the potential magnitude of the current threat.

Self-Designed.

individual to commit a dangerous act, based upon "FILMing" their past and present violent and/or dangerous threats and actions, within the contexts of their social groups' policies, and against a known set of risk factors.

We all belong to a minimum of three social groups: family or surrogate family; peer groups, which are often school, work, recreational clubs, and the like; and greater societal contexts, such as larger organizations, cities, counties, states, and nations. They can also be gangs, clicks, church groups, and so on. The social groups the POI belongs to each have their own sets of values, morays, rules, laws, dress codes, and other expectations by which every member of that group is expected to abide. For example, a drug cartel's rules will be substantially different than a church youth group's rules. Hence, the POI's social group contexts can provide enormous insights into their dangerousness risk. Remember, the greater the number, the greater the frequency, and especially the greater the variety of past violent events and weapons to which they've been exposed, the higher their propensity to act out the threatened violence.

The Federal Commission on School Violence Signs of Increasing Risk comprises two short and simple DRA tools: behaviors, risk factors, grievances, resentments, and changes in behaviors, risk factors, grievances, and resentments. They are easily remembered using the acronyms BRGR ("Burger") and CBRGR ("Cheeseburger").

Behaviors are the way in which a person acts in response to particular situations or stimuli. Risk factors are a known set of factors used to determine the risk level for any person at any time to behave dangerously. The top ten risk factors for behaving dangerously are sufficient to guide one's next steps in assessing, reducing, or even eliminating the person's risk.

In order to proceed, it is critical to accurately know and appreciate the meaning of grievances and resentments:

1. Grievances are *real or imagined wrongs* or other causes for complaints, especially unfair treatment.
2. Resentments are the very complex *emotions* one feels when they are wronged or when they perceive they were wronged, real or imagined. Resentments are a combination of the emotions of painful bitterness, fury, rage, acrimony, malice, and annoyance felt when one has been wronged or even just perceives they were wronged, *even if it's not real.*

Grievances and resentments permeate everything about dangerousness risk.

Thousands of retrospective analyses of POIs and the surrounding circumstances of past violent, suicidal, and even avoidable accidents, called forensic psychiatric autopsies, and prospective evaluations of persons expressing feelings of behaving dangerously toward others, those having suicidal thoughts or behaviors, and even those experiencing avoidable accidents reveal the top ten risk factors for behaving dangerously. The top ten risk factors can easily be remembered using the acronym "SAD PERSONS."

When Dr. Kevin Smith initially created the SAD PERSONS program for the U.S. military to stop the suicide epidemic occurring at that time, he did so by conducting forensic psychiatric autopsies. Those autopsies revealed 10 common risk factors for the cases under review. More importantly, autopsies revealed that numerous soldiers and civilians close to the deceased had observed one or two of those risk factors but wrote them off as nothing, even though they were disturbed by those actions. There was no designated reporting scheme or program for addressing concerns, which is the key to prevention.

Dr. Smith presented his recommendation to the U.S. Army Command: Train everyone in the SAD PERSONS acronym and dispense wallet-sized cards listing those risk factors on the front. On the back, place a pyramid displaying each community member's chain of reporting to ensure the risk factors for the POI were systematically organized. The military is excellent in organizing a chain of command to ensure nothing falls through the cracks. This was an attempt to use this system to prevent a suicide epidemic, as well as other mental health issues.

For active duty personnel their reporting paradigm was their chain of command with which they were already familiar. For the staff and students of the Department of Defense Dependents Schools (DODDS), the schools provided the training, and their administrator would report the data to the commander. Why? It's because one distressed family member can distress other members, which could result in the death of active duty personnel and/ or their dependents.

One division alone consisted of approximately 35,000 people, including dependents and civilian contractors. How can that many people in one division, let alone multiple divisions, be trained in the SAD PERSONS prevention program? Simple. Train the trainer. Keep in mind that this program started back when the only presentation methods available were chalkboards, overhead projectors, and transparencies. Computers, the internet, and cell phones make training everyone in today's world much more practical and expeditious.

Within one year, suicide deaths had dropped to zero and accidental deaths had dropped dramatically. Homicides were rare at that time. These trainings were repeated every year.

When suspicion arises that an active duty soldier has developed an elevated risk, the chain of command passes the data up the chain to the appropriate level so they could be referred to mental health professionals.

It soon became evident to Dr. Smith and his team that the same risk factors applied to externalized violence and accidental deaths. The military in turn made changes to reflect the new observations.

The SAD PERSONS acronym that created this program is as follows:

S = Sex; males are ten times more likely to complete suicide than females.
A = Aged between10 and 29 years.
D = Distressed mentally, which is not limited to diagnosable mental illness.
P = Previous exposure to suicidal behavior in self or others.
E = Ethanol, which is a placeholder in one's memory for alcohol and/or drug use.
R = Rational thinking loss from any cause.

S = Social support system lacking or perceived to be lacking, which includes being bullied.

O = Organized plan, meaning who, what, where, when, and/or how. Any one of these elements must be considered as an emergency to be evaluated by experts.

N = No spouse, significant other, or solid attachment to an adult, which itself is a very bad prognostic indicator.

S = Serious, chronic, and/or terminal illness.

KEY IDEAS TO REMEMBER

Dangerousness risk assessment is a very useful tool for assessing a person's risk to commit a dangerous act. They may externalize their angst against other people or property, or turn their emotions inward and target their violence against themselves through suicidal actions. Externalized violence and internalized violence meld with one another as most people externalizing their violence expect to die while doing so. Most active shooters create a situation where law enforcement will take a kill shot, or they take their own life rather than be arrested.

The overarching goal is to intervene prior to the POI acting out their grievances and resentments in a violent manner. A common language for addressing POIs is utilized by mental health professionals, law enforcement, behavioral assessment units, the FBI, Secret Service, U.S. Department of Homeland Security, and others. Two of the most powerful tools used are BRGR and CBRGR, as they specifically relate to profiling potential aggresses. These tools help us remember the critical facets: behaviors, risk factors, grievances, and resentments, and changes in behaviors, risk factors, grievances, and resentments.

The meaning of grievances and resentments must be memorized, so they're in the forefront of one's mind all the time:

Grievances are *real or imagined wrongs* or other causes for complaints, especially unfair treatment.

Resentments are the very complex *emotions* one feels when wronged or perceive they were wronged, real or imagined. Resentments are a combination of the emotions of painful bitterness, fury, rage, acrimony, malice and annoyance felt when one has been wronged or just perceives they were wronged, *even if it's not real.*

Another very useful tool in the tool box for assessing dangerousness risk, which dovetails into BRGR and CBRGR, is the SAD PERSONS acronym. It serves to remind us of the *top ten risk factors* for behaving violently toward others, oneself, and property. Remember, the first "R" in BRGR stands for "risk factors," so SAD PERSONS completes the tool box.

Keep in mind that not all POIs will exhibit all the 10 characteristics in SAD PERSONS. Age and sex are static risk factors, meaning they are what they are, which basically is an indicator that males are more dangerous in general than females. However, even one of the remaining 8 risk factors can tip the scales over to the "concerned" side, and at a minimum that POI needs a professional mental health evaluation and possibly a law enforcement assessment of their previous exposure to weapons and violence.

Chapter 7

SAD PERSONS

Males have ten times the propensity as females to behave violently against others or property.

When someone exhibits one or more of SAD PERSONS risk factors, it is time to get some professional help so that a DRA may be conducted. The exceptions are the two static, or unchangeable, factors: age and sex. Either or both do not establish risk without at least one of the dynamic factors.

The risk factors for externalized violence, internalized violence (suicide), and accidents are very similar and are often identical to one another. They are described here.

S = Sex: Males have ten times the propensity as females to behave violently against others or property. In the United States, school mass shooters have thus far all been male. There have already been some reported incidences of females perpetrating acts of school violence against multiple victims using knives, but so far they have not been perpetrators of mass school shootings. Males are also more likely to behave recklessly and carelessly, increasing their likelihood of accidents and accidental death.

As with violence, males are ten times more likely than females to complete their suicide. Males more often complete their suicide, because they use more lethal means, such as irreversible hanging, gunshot to the head or torso, or jumping off a very high platform. Females have historically attempted suicide more often than males, but have used less lethal means, such as overdoses or superficial cutting of the wrists. They also tend to avoid using means that could leave them significantly or unacceptably disfigured, such as jumping or gunshot to the head. That being said, over the last several years, female suicide completions have been rising dramatically as females have been getting more and more aggressive in their attempts and their means.

A = Age: To date, school shooters have been between the ages of 10 and 29. This comes as no surprise, given the age range for students in school, including those in college and those pursuing advanced degrees.

Interestingly, FBI crime data statistics show that over 90% of all arrests in the United States are also in the age group of 12 to 29, the highest number of arrests being between 16 and 22, with a maximum peak in the bell-shaped curve at age 18. By age 30, arrest rates drop off dramatically.

The age range for most suicide attempts and completions is also 12 to 29, although the lower age level has been steadily falling *below* 10 years old for the last 10 years or so. There is a second peak for suicide in the 60s for the elderly that fail to embrace charity toward others and instead fall into loneliness and despair.

The peak age range for most accidental deaths is also from 12 to 29 years, due to the volume and intensity of reckless, careless, distracted, intentionally illegal, and risk-taking behaviors.

D = Distressed Mentally From Any Cause:

Mental distress does not just include diagnosable mental illness. It can also refer to anything that stresses us as human beings, such as being bullied, sleep deprivation, financial worries, and so on. Mental distress must be assessed and understood from the perspective of the person feeling distressed. Although human beings generally have more in common with one another than they do not have in common, not everyone responds to the same stressors in life to similar degrees and in similar ways. This may be a useful starting point, but simply judging another person's mental distress from one's own perspective can miss the brewing crisis beneath the surface. The best policy is to get them to tell you what their stressors are and how those stressors are affecting them.

One should also appreciate that it's a mistake to presume a person with mental illness is imminently dangerous. In fact, people with diagnosed mental illness who are compliant with their treatment and their medications are no more dangerous than anyone else. Those studies have been done and replicated many times over. However, mentally ill persons who are not complaint with their treatment and medications can become violent toward themselves, others, and/or property.

Family members and friends of mentally ill persons can do so much to keep that person from potentially becoming violent by being supportive and encouraging them to stay compliant with their treatment regimen. Anyone who believes that a friend or loved one is not compliant can and should notify local community mental health services or that person's treatment provider. Mental health providers cannot share confidential treatment information without the patient's consent. In fact, they will probably say something like: "I can neither confirm nor deny that the person you name has ever been my client." However, they can always receive information and concerns from other sources, and hopefully will then discuss that information and those concerns with the patient.

Asking someone you know or care about if they have been thinking about hurting themselves or someone else *does not* put the idea into their heads, nor does it cause them to act on the idea. People who are thinking about suicide or homicide are doing so because *they feel totally helpless and hopeless* about their situation changing. They desperately want someone to perceive their emotional pain, listen, and help. Getting them to share their thoughts or feelings of harming themselves or others is the best first step to preventing a violent act, externalized toward others or internalized against themselves. And remember, *those who externalize their violence prepare for their own death.*

It is very useful when assessing mental distress to ask about the top six stressors in life. Five of them are death of a loved one, divorce, moving, major illness, and job loss or financial difficulties. Due to a research article published in the December 2018 edition of the American Psychiatric Association Journal, a sixth top stressor is added to this list: parental mental distress can cause mental distress in their children that will very likely result in acting out behaviors in school.

Accidents are very common among the mentally distressed. Mental distress interferes with focus, vigilance, concentration, acuity, recall, and alertness. These are all vital brain functions that keep each of us safe every day. Mental distress can become severely disabling and ultimately result in an accident or multiple accidents.

P = Previous Exposure to Violence, Weapons or Suicide: The greater the number, the frequency, and especially the variety of violent events previously exposed to, the higher the risk of behaving violently in the present. Likewise, the greater the number, the frequency, and especially the variety of weapons exposure, the higher the risk of behaving violently in the present.

Previous exposure to weapons and violence is rampant among mass school shooters. Most of us are surprised, shocked, and horrified every time we have another school shooting and eventually learn that someone in the shooter's family bought weapons and ammunition for their child and trained their child how to use those weapons.

Regarding mass shootings in schools, assault rifles have been the most commonly used weapons, followed by automatic and semiautomatic handguns. Knives have been the third most commonly used class of weapons, and improvised explosive devices (IED), such as pipe bombs, have been much less common.

Exposure to previous suicidal behavior by the person themselves or someone else raises their risk of suicide. This includes exposure to suicidal behavior by people one does not personally know.

On April 5, 1994, at the age of 27, the very popular Nirvana grunge singer, Kurt Cobain, died of a self-inflicted 20-gauge shotgun shot to his head. In the five days that followed, about a dozen students from one high school in New York State were admitted to the psychiatric unit of the local hospital after attempting suicide themselves, creating a copycat suicide epidemic. None of them personally knew the singer, and fortunately none of them succeeded. The take-home message here is that it is not necessary that the POI personally know the deceased to be dangerously influenced by their actions.

E = Ethanol: Alcohol serves as a placeholder for remembering that alcohol and drug use are another of the top ten risk factors for violence, suicide, and accidents. The take-home message here is that even recreational use of mind-altering substances, let alone abuse of them, increases everyone's likelihood of behaving dangerously, suicidally, and recklessly. In fact, just being in the midst of users can lead to disinhibition of the nonuser.

Many of these mind-altering substances are often stored in medicine cabinets, where children and their friends can access them whenever they want. *Keep all medications secured at all times!* Demonstrating to your children that you trust them by not securing your medications is foolish. Don't do it! Teaching your children trust can be accomplished in many ways that are much safer. Besides, children may still want to impress their friends, or demonstrate that they're cool, or their friends will simply take advantage of the open access provided, and you will be held legally and psychologically liable for whatever happens next.

"Pill parties" have become a recent rage among kids and young adults. They obtain any and every pill they can find in their homes and bring them to a party site, where all the pills are dumped into a communal bowl to be accessed at will by everyone in attendance, along with alcoholic beverages also obtained from home. These parties are highly dangerous due to potentially toxic combinations of unknown substances and potentially deadly substances alone.

Many substances can increase violent, suicidal, and accidental behaviors and urges.

R = Rational Thinking Loss: Irrationality from any cause increases one's risk of violence, suicide, and accidents. This includes such "normal" things as sleep deprivation, stress, or even adolescence itself. Our brains, including our frontal lobes where executive functions such as rational thinking reside, are not fully matured until our mid-twenties. Additionally, hormones are the chemical drive behind many essential bodily functions and regulatory systems. Those hormones are in flux through adolescence and into early adulthood. They only begin to settle down around the mid-twenties.

It should come as no surprise that the FBI's arrest rates peak at age 18 and die down dramatically after age 29. Recklessness, carelessness, risk taking, believing one can get away with forbidden conduct, and intentionally choosing to break the law are common in this age group. The frequency and intensity of these behaviors begin to rise around 11 to 12 years old, are highest between 16 and 22 years, and peak at 18 years of age. It is this very reckless, careless, risky, forbidden, and/or illegal conduct that results in 16- to 22-year-olds having the highest arrest rate in the United States, high suicide rates, and also very high rates of accidental deaths.

S = Strong Social Support System Lacking: It is critical to appreciate that the lack of social support, especially the lack of a solid attachment to an adult, is a very, very bad prognostic indicator. That child or person will have difficulties with human bonding, socializing, being an integral member of social groups, and being able to truly appreciate the nature of a human-to-human relationship. Strong social support plays a critical role in the individual's growth into a healthy, happy, and productive life. After all, humans are social animals by nature. Those who have little or no loving, concerned, caring interactions with their parents, relatives, nonfamilial adults, even peers and schoolmates will struggle to develop strong social support systems. They may also be a bullied student.

Everyone must keep a vigilant eye out for the marginalized and the loners. To do this everyone must work diligently at making sure these people are integrated into the social network of the organization, especially schools. Classmates should be encouraged to reach out and invite marginalized children into their groups, leading by example for the other students. In New York State, SEL is now part of every school district's curriculum that receives federal and state funding. SEL specifically espouses these ideals of inclusion and support.

Lastly, it's very important to remember the adage, "Keep your friends close and your enemies closer." It used to be the case that school leaders were directed to send the potentially dangerous, threatening students home and get them a home tutor. That's no longer considered the best practice. If the student is sent home, both the school and law enforcement have no easy way of monitoring and tracking the student's thinking, behaviors, emotional condition, and other useful observational data important to the student's well-being and the safety of the school and other students. The best practice is to make sure those students are not left marginalized but rather welcomed by their peers and teachers into the integrated social spheres.

The FBI now recommends that the student stay in school with frequent checks with the school administration and with a teacher or teachers with whom they have a good relationship. This approach provides much more opportunity to uncover early signs and symptoms of possible emotional deterioration and increasing dangerousness risk, and to provide corrective intervention. School resource officers (SROs) can be very helpful and extremely good at this.

While at the topic of SROs, it absolutely must be underscored just how valuable and mission critical SROs can be. Observations have shown that the very students most at risk of acting out, staging pranks, or behaving recklessly and carelessly are the ones that gravitate most intensely to the SROs. Strong bonds often quickly get established and strengthen over time. The at-risk student now has a mentor that they respect, probably even comes to cherish, and possibly the first adult that has demonstrated a sincere respect and empathic appreciation of them. Do not minimize or overlook these amazing SROs who choose to help these kids find their way through a solid relationship with an adult.

O = Organized Plans: Plans developed by the POI, which include even *just one of who, where, when or how*, or applied to a violent, suicidal and/or accidental risk must be considered an emergency to be immediately assessed, preferably by trained professionals in law enforcement and mental health. However, school administrators will most likely be on the front line when this crisis unfolds, and will have to execute their protocols as per their established plan.

N = No Spouse or Significant Other: This risk factor is of special concern because it illustrates a lack of attachment. Adolescence through young adulthood is a critical period for transitioning one's primary focus of love from the nuclear family to a specially selected peer group member. If the person does not make this transition successfully, social isolation and grievances are likely to develop. Resentments will then likely emerge and fester, which can lead to a very dangerous and volatile situation. Watch for the loners and reach out to them. Remember once again that *lack of a solid attachment to an adult is a very, very bad prognostic indicator.*

S = Serious, Chronic, or Varied Violent Behaviors: The more serious, the more chronic, and especially the more varied the violent behaviors, the higher the risk of behaving violently now.

Serious, chronic or terminal illnesses raise the risk of suicide. The more serious, the more chronic, especially the more varied the suicidal behaviors in the past, the higher the risk of behaving suicidally at this juncture. This can be major to minor ailments, so don't be misled into believing it has to be cancer, kidney failure, or an inoperable brain tumor. A U.S. Army sergeant presented to sick call repeatedly complaining of an intractable and "very painful" toothache. After six weeks of trying unsuccessfully to get relief from his pain by going repeatedly to the dentist asking for help, he lamented he had gotten no pain relief, gave up hope, shot himself in the head, and died in the dentist's office on base.

Very notably, as of the fall of 2019, there is a suicide epidemic with American youth that is spiraling out of control. According to the president of the

American Psychiatric Association (APA), much more mental health services must be urgently made available in order to curb this epidemic.

KEY IDEAS TO REMEMBER

There is not one single authoritative profile of an active shooter. However, the following profile is very close, and anyone exhibiting two or more of the characteristics discussed below must be considered a POI.

The POI is a male between the ages of 10 and 29. He has had exposure to weapons and violence and may currently be using or abusing drugs and/or alcohol. He is challenged in his ability to think rationally and has isolated himself from family, friends, and/or coworkers. As such, he lacks an attachment to another person and tends to be a loner. Without naming any names, he has recently posted on social media his feelings of rage at those around him. His demeanor is encroaching on a serious and violent side. Much of his time is spent planning an act to get even with those whom he feels have wronged him.

The goal is to prevent the above profiled POI from finishing the plan and acting it out. The manner in which we can stop this is through notifying law enforcement or school leaders of a concern for a person's behavior so that a DRA may be conducted. Recognizing the warning signs and acting upon them will save a life, or more.

Chapter 8

Why This Age Group?

When language fails, violence becomes the language.

—Elie Wiesel

Why is the 12 to 29 years age group so vulnerable to behaving dangerously? A plethora of clues can be found in the biopsychosocial model, group process dynamics, basic personality growth theory, FBI arrest rates, causes of death, evolution of school disciplinary problems, and special issues with bullying.

The biopsychosocial model: What follows is just a glimpse of the complex volumes of what goes on biologically, psychologically, and sociologically in this age group. In reality, it's much worse.

Biologically, humans are incompletely developed during their teens, into their early twenties, and with some human aspects even up to around 30 years of age. Hormones are churning if not raging, which alone can cause irritability, interfere with sleep-wake cycle, escalate conflicts, and result in thunderstorms of mood instability. Fortunately, these unstable hormonal patterns start settling down sometime in the twenties, which is the same age we now know that the brain itself fully matures. Until then, humans must also deal with immature areas of the brain responsible for sound judgment and sensible decisions.

Psychologically, adolescents and young adults must overcome those thunderstorms of mood instability. They are also inexperienced, immature, and impulsive. Wisdom has not fully matured, which may lead to bad decisions, and this in turn can result in impulsively reckless, careless, and aggressive behaviors. They struggle with self-esteem, self-awareness, and sexual issues, including sexual preferences and behaviors. Basically, everything about them is in an uproar.

Sociologically, there are two important, age-specific developmental objectives that must be successfully achieved between the ages of 18 and 23: separate from one's nuclear family and find membership in one's own peer group, meaning settling into searches for and trials with potential life partners. Ultimately, the typical goal is to find "the one." Achieving these two objectives is often very laden with conflict.

Group Process Dynamics: Why are joining groups and leaving groups so inherently conflict laden? Group dynamics is the main stage for this developmental objective.

A *group* is defined as two or more people coming together for common goals. Couples, families, friends, co-workers, peers, sport teams, organizations, and businesses are all examples of groups.

There are four basic, simplified phases to group process. Phases are the various stages a group must successfully navigate together in order to ultimately complete the common group purpose and move on to the next stage. The four phases are shown in figure 8.1.

Each phase varies in length and difficulty. Regardless of the difficulty of each phase, it is evident that conflict plays a major role in the dynamics of each group.

Group process occurs every day, everywhere, and generally without our awareness that it is occurring. Human beings are social animals, which makes it virtually impossible for us to avoid social interactions. The next time a group of students is considering entering into a group task, watch, listen,

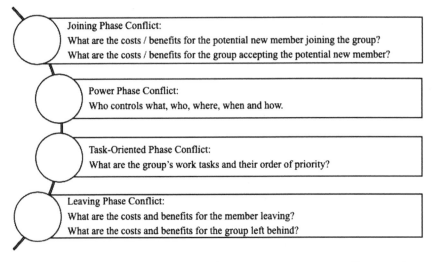

Figure 8.1   The Four Phases Associated with Group Process. *Source*: Self-Designed, MS Word.

and learn. There will be a leader, a notetaker, an organizer, a creator, a lazy nonparticipant, and possibly even a stick-in-the-mud. Observe what it takes to engage the reluctant members in the task. Group dynamic management is a highly useful skill to get students engaged with their peers. This is a skill that if practiced today, could very well save lives tomorrow.

Erik Erikson's Basic Theory of Personality Growth: This theory provides a simplified overview of the human personality spectrum over a lifetime and helps explain how the 12 to 29 years age span is so critical. Erikson identified several stages of life, which when each is successfully achieved is called a potency, and when not successfully achieved is called an impotency.

Stage one, for example, spans birth to about 12 to 18 months of age and deals with the struggle between hope and basic trust and despair and basic mistrust. How do humans learn hope and basic trust? When hungry, infants cry and someone feeds them. When uncomfortable from a soiled diaper, they cry and someone cleans them up. When they fall down and get hurt, they cry and someone comforts them. When they cannot sleep, they cry and someone rocks them back to sleep. Through these interactions they are learning that a cry for help will bring comfort, a smiling face, even joy. If these human interactions do not occur, or occur too infrequently, infants develop depression, where they assume a state of despair and basic mistrust. This is the first human experience with trusting in and relying upon others to support, nurture, care for, and love us.

With each incomplete achievement of a life stage goal one accumulates more and more impotencies. A quick look at the impotencies of the first six stages of development reveals where this path leads (figure 8.2).

People who missed out on some, most, or all of these potencies grow up with difficulty or inability to enjoy a solid attachment to an adult or in some

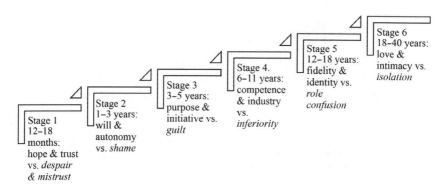

Figure 8.2 Six Stages That Provide the Basis for Understanding Why the Periods of Adolescence and Young Adulthood Are So Crucial for Interpersonal Social Development. *Source*: Self-Designed.

cases to their peers. It should not surprise anyone that people who accumulate many elements of these impotencies—despair, mistrust, shame, guilt, inferiority, role confusion, and isolation—either become socially isolated or attach to other similar and like-minded resentful people who also accumulate real or perceived grievances.

These first six stages provide the basis for understanding why the periods of adolescence and young adulthood are so crucial for interpersonal social development. If one fails to sufficiently achieve each stage, they end up on a spiraling path that prevents successful maturation into adulthood. A few examples of people who failed to successfully navigate the stages of human development include Erik Harris and Dillon Klebold from Columbine and Nikolas Cruz from Marjory Stoneman High School.

Given the social development issues associated with this age group, it is not surprising to see why the FBI are particularly interested in them.

FBI Arrest Rates: FBI arrest rates have been maintained for decades and provide another source of insight into the problem of school violence. The FBI composite rates show the number of arrests occurring per 100,000 per year by ages of those arrested. The highest arrest rates occur between the ages of 16 and 22, with a sharp rise from 16 to 18 years of age and the highest peak at 18. This peak at 18 years of age is followed by a gradual but significant decline from 18 to 30 years.

Leading Causes of Death: The leading causes of death for ages 12 to 29 are shown in figure 8.3.

Motor Vehicle Accidents (MVAs) are the number one cause of death in this age group, with MVAs due to texting while driving being the top subcategory. The second highest subcategory is MVAs with a teen driver and one or more teenage passengers, but without a parent or legal guardian in the car.

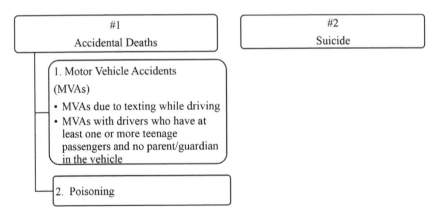

Figure 8.3   Accidental Deaths and Suicide Are the Leading Causes of Death for 12- to 29-year-olds. *Source:* Self-Designed.

Both accidental and intentional poisonings are the second leading group of accidental deaths in this age group. Accidental poisonings include such things as drinking a jar of liquid thought to be ethanol alcohol, when it's actually propyl alcohol or windshield washing fluid (polyethylene glycol). Intentional poisonings include lacing one's marijuana joints with embalming fluid or swallowing Tide Pods on a dare.

School Misconduct Evolution: Misbehavior has evolved over the decades with some eye-opening revelations. In the 1940s studies were done looking at the top disciplinary problems facing schools. They include talking out of turn, chewing gum, making noise, running in the hall, cutting in line, dress code violations, and littering. Studies completed in more recent years reveal the top disciplinary problems facing our schools, which include bullying, drug and alcohol abuse, rape, robbery, assault, and murder. This data clearly represent a significant and dangerous shift in "school misconduct."

Bullying has become a special concern: One common denominator of many students who act out or try to self-harm is that they were bullied or they perceived themselves to have been bullied. It's easy to jump to the conclusion that it must be because the bullied child has a much more difficult time of integrating socially with their peers, developing normal self-esteem, perhaps participating in sports, and so on. This may be true but is now not the only truth.

There is now *anatomical evidence* that bullying causes actual brain damage in key areas of the child's brain. It's been proven that kids who are bullied have a higher risk of behavioral and psychological problems than those who have not experienced bullying.

In an effort to address the growing epidemic of bullying in New York State, the state passed DASA in September 2010. This law ensured that disrespectful acts in schools had to be addressed and formally reported annually to the NYS Department of Education. It had lofty goals, many which were not achieved, but it did bring the topic of bullying in schools to the forefront and forced school personnel to address the issue.

Of interest is what caused the uptick in bullying in schools? Many argue the increased prevalence of social media, cell phones, and social apps are the cause. Students today are living in a virtual fishbowl as many of their interactions and actions are recorded and posted for their peers to see. Not being invited to a party in the past may have been known by a few people. Now "You are not invited" posts clearly point out that you are not part of the in-group. As noted earlier, one stressor for students is the lack of a social support system. A sense of belonging that is broken can have a significant impact on a child's psyche.

The December 27, 2018, edition of the *Journal of Molecular Psychiatry* published a significant study demonstrating that teens who are "often" bullied suffer "observable and measurable losses of brain volume." In this study, 700 teens across Europe were repeatedly evaluated from 14 through 19 years of age with serial brain scans, serial comprehensive psychological testing, and serial psychological evaluations.

The study reported that 37 out of the 700 kids studied were often and chronically bullied over five years or less. All 37 of the chronically bullied kids developed "observable & measurable losses of brain volume" in two key areas deep in the brain, known as the left caudate and left putamen nuclei. *Additionally, all 37 of the chronically bullied kids developed the emotional processing problems of hyperactivity, anxiety, and depression.*

The fact that the brain volume losses occurred in the left nuclei is significant in that over 90% of human beings worldwide are left hemisphere dominant. Hemisphere dominance is completely different from handedness. The significance of the left hemisphere dominance is that those two nuclei in the left hemisphere are the ones that control the very vital functions of: attention; motivation; learning; communication skills; approach-attachment behaviors (human bonding); memory storage, access, and processing; using information from past experiences to influence future actions and decisions; and controlling body limb posture. In addition, the seat of obsessive-compulsive disorder (OCD) appears to be in this area of the brain as well. What is not yet known is whether or not the tissue lost in these two left-sided nuclei can regrow. A full understanding of just how the bullying victim's mental and behavioral risks emerge and evolve is in its infancy, but it holds much promise for further understanding of its full impact. Further research is ongoing.

Because of these findings, the potential liability concerns for schools and school districts have rapidly become a top priority focus for their insurers.

Individuals aged 12 to 29 years lack full brain development and as such have an increased propensity for acting dangerously. This age group struggles with controlling urges, are often careless, are prone to make bad decisions, and tend to be aggressive. These actions alone make this age group challenging. Add in that many have access to weapons, and the age group takes on a whole new level of challenging.

The debate will continue regarding our Second Amendment Right to Bear Arms. What is not heard in these debates are the following:

- Persons aged 16 through 22 have biologically incomplete brains and are in the highest age group for arrests in the United States.
- Psychologically, they have mood instability; immaturity; impulsiveness; poor judgment; reckless, and careless and aggressive behaviors. They struggle with self-esteem, self-awareness, and sexual maturation and choices.
- Decades of data about FBI arrest rates show the 16 to 22 age group has the highest rate of arrests, and those arrest rates don't fall back to baseline until 30 years of age.

- We know that the top causes of death for this same age group are accidents, with number one being MVAs caused by texting while driving. The number two cause is a teen driver with more than one teen passenger and without a parent or legal guardian in the vehicle with them.
- The second leading accidental death for the same age group is poisoning, both accidental and intentional, due to bad decisions.
- School disciplinary problems for 16- to 22-year-olds have evolved, with the top ones now being bullying, drug and alcohol abuse, rape, robbery, assault, and murder.

Given the above data, from a professional forensic perspective, this begs for studies about various strategies for licensing firearms, especially automatic and semiautomatic ones, to our most immature, recklessly, carelessly and illegally behaving societal age group. This age group easily finds individuals who may fester grievances and resentments that eventually solidify into a foundation of justification for threatening, assaultive, even annihilative actions.

KEY IDEAS TO REMEMBER

The FBI are very interested in the 12 to 29 age group, because of the damage and social uproar they can cause. The reasons for their reckless, careless, and impulsive behaviors are found in the biopsychosocial model of human development combined with group process dynamics of human-to-human interactions. Personality growth, or more specifically lack of growth and immaturity, result in the accumulation of the personality impotencies of despair, mistrust, shame, guilt, inferiority, role confusion, and isolation. Past school and mall shooters have accumulated most, if not all, of these impotencies in their development.

The combination of FBI arrest rates and known primary causes of death in this age group points again to a very reckless, careless, and impulsive population, inherently making them more dangerous as a group. And finally, we now know that "often bullied" victims have visible and measurable brain tissue losses in key areas of their brains that contribute to their emotional, social, cognitive, and learning difficulties on an anatomical level.

There is still much more to learn, and, in turn, much to do, to turn the tide of bullying among children.

Chapter 9

Risk Factors and Dynamic Mental Health

What is the likelihood that the POI will indeed harm themselves or others? Interestingly enough, DRA for homicide and suicide are the same.

Mental health has been discussed in a variety of manners throughout this book because it is deeply intertwined with threat and DRAs. It is imperative that everyone understand that mental health is not synonymous with mentally ill. Mental health refers to the stressors that a person is struggling with. Stressors may manifest themselves into attitudes and behaviors that may in turn cause a DRA to take place.

Mental health issues are of critical importance as a majority of active shooters exhibited this stressor. Some of the common stressors are depression, anxiety, perceived or real bullying, paranoia, grievances, and resentments. More often than not these stressors are internalized and professional help is shunned or rarely provided. Lack of professional help may be due to the denial of having any issues or possibly because the warning signs were missed. One thing is for certain, the mental health of the individuals who acted aggressively was in distress.

The FBI studied active shooter cases between 2000 and 2013 and found that a majority of the shooters experienced mental stressors prior to their acts of aggression. Their stressors were associated with where they worked as well as with peers and peer groups and resulted in obvious observable behaviors. Behaviors exhibited by former active shooters left peers and coworkers uneasy about their behavior. This is significant as it means that recognition of these behaviors can quickly escalate a DRA to take place and quite possibly thwart a potential shooting.

Active shooters have internalized grievances that were very personal to them. They do not rage against large organizations or ideology. Rather, they have grievances that are very personal to their life. They may have a grievance with a classmate, failed to earn a spot on an athletic team, been subjected to ongoing bullying, or have an issue with a romantic relationship. Their stressors can often create a desire to commit suicide as their brains and maturity are not at the point where rational decisions can be made. Instead, grievances are harbored and internalized as resentments. Resentments grow to the point where the person's behavior and demeanor changes.

Changes in behavior are not something that take place just before the aggressive act. Rather, the grievances and resentments harbored by the individual causes stress. This stress begins to affect their behavior and demeanor as early as two years prior to the final act of violence. The issue festers and grows. Research notes that every single active shooter experienced stressors in the final weeks and days leading up to the attack. It is during this critical time, when their behavior is changing that situational awareness must kick in. On average, active shooters displayed four to five concerning behaviors over time according to the FBI study (2018).

Behaviors of interest are part of the previously identified SAD PERSONS acronym. SAD PERSONS is an easy way to remember the top ten risk factors for behaving violently, which was previously discussed.

SAD PERSONS assists the DRA threat team in assessing a POI. It's also very useful for schools to use when conducting spot checks on students exhibiting possible signs of distress. They are not organized according to their significance in assessing risk. In fact, the average reader need not concern themselves with learning, let alone memorizing, their order of significance, because the overriding purpose of SAD PERSONS (see figure 9.1) is to help individuals recognize potential elevated risk factors and then funnel the information up the pyramid of expertise in the DRA team so that the risk factor gets consolidated. Each risk factor alone may not ring a bell, but a consolidation of them will most certainly RING the bell. This alone is a huge leap forward in prevention of violence. Always funnel risk factors up your pyramid of expertise.

It is not imperative that all ten elements be evident when assessing the risk factors.

Sometimes an individual will only exhibit a few risk factors, but the severity of some of the risks may be extreme.

There is much to be said about following your gut. Should there be disagreement when conducting the assessments, always err on the side of taking it too seriously. It is far easier to apologize and make amends than to explain to parents, colleagues, and friends why innocent people were placed

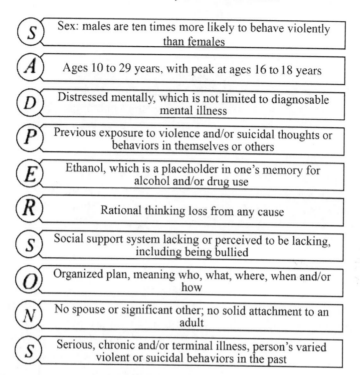

Figure 9.1 Ten Potential Elevated Risk Factors to Be Aware of When Spot Checking for Signs of Distress in Students. *Source*: Self-Designed.

in harm's way. Those closest to the potential shooter have the highest likelihood to recognize changes in behavior. A new normal needs to kick in where concerning behaviors, even those observed by friends, family, and co-workers, need to be reported. Missed interventions significantly increase the propensity for violence.

To assist schools in identifying at-risk students early the incorporation of mental health programs within the schools has dramatically increased. Through county, state, and federal assistance with funding, schools are now able to provide mental health screenings and services to students from pre-kindergarten through grade 12. Schools now have access to mental health counselors and there is always lobbying for more state and federal funding to increase these services.

Additionally, character education continues to grow in terms of its incorporation in the school's curriculum by including social-emotional learning. Enhancing on the decades-old character education piece, new programming is being developed to address many societal ills. These include restorative justice, positive behavior intervention services (PBIS), and real restitution.

Character education helps teach the soft skills of respect, conflict resolution, relationship-building, responsibility, and anti-bullying.

The SAD PERSONS risk assessment acronym helps to determine if the child is distraught over issues with peers, family, or society, or if they have adjusted. It was previously described in detail in chapter 7. For those with stressors in their lives, a good week today may not remain in a couple of weeks. Given any type of volatility it is crucial to bring in mental health experts.

When making an assessment of a person's mental distress, it is useful to explore the top five stressors in life, which are listed in figure 9.2.

If the POI is a child, it is important to remember that the parents' distress in their own lives will cause significant distress in the child's life, so much so that acting out in school is expected.

KEY IDEAS TO REMEMBER

Mental Health issues are of critical importance in recognizing potential impending elevated dangerous risk that can lead to the emergence of an actual shooting or worse. The signs of increasing risk will manifest themselves as described in the SAD PERSONS acronym, so use it. Rely on it! This chapter has laid out what can be done to identify and help the emerging *person of interest* and provide them with person-specific interventions and assistance.

Providing successful mental health intervention is not rocket science. Each and every one of us has experienced many if not all of the trials and tribulations the current POI is dealing with. Do not hesitate to use your own experiences in life to guide your efforts with this person, since at least 80% of the time you'll be spot on with your first attempt. If the person would prefer

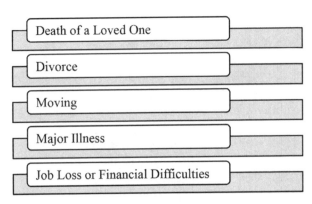

Figure 9.2 **Top Five Mental Health Stressors.** *Source*: Self-Designed.

working with someone else, by all means make that happen. This is not a turf war, it is a necessary action that will improve and possibly save a life.

What is very well established scientifically is that the single most important factor in achieving successful mental health treatment is the development of a strong, trusting relationship with the provider—a bond. The average person has the capacity to be that strong and trusted "provider." This is all about human empathy and compassion. Also, use the mental health resources available in the school and its community to provide this troubled person with any additional services they may need to restore their sense of security, stability, and serenity.

Chapter 10

Learning from Real-Life Experiences

I've waited my whole life for just this one day.

—Mall Shooter

The following case studies are real-life examples that occurred in New York State. Some names and locations have been changed to protect the identity of the individuals, their families, their schools, and their communities. Otherwise the facts of the cases are solid. As you read through each case take the time to ask yourself what you would do to help the individual before things cross from bad to dangerous. Working each case together in small groups is an excellent way to study and learn from them.

Additionally, ask yourself what you would do if you were in the vicinity when the violence occurred. Lastly, please make a vow to yourself to be vigilantly aware of those around you. *When something seems to be off, it probably is off.* Go with your gut and investigate it or get help to investigate the situation. Lives depend upon you acting on your gut.

As noted in previous chapters, there are simple, useful tools for implementing the DRA, which are briefly listed here for convenience:

- BRGRs and CBRGRs
- Propensity, both retrospective and prospective
- Adolescents and young adults openly and accurately indicate their own violence plans
- Social memberships
- SADPERSONS top ten risk factors

There is no set calculus for summing up one's findings into a numerical risk. However, methodically going through the risk factors will provide a very useful gestalt for concluding where the person's risk level stands. Assigning levels of "Normal, Low, Medium, High" will suffice. This gestalt then guides the decisions regarding interventions. Err on the side of caution. If you're not sure if the level is Medium or High, call it High.

CASE 1: *JOHN AND JANE GO DOWN HILL*

Family Court placed Jane with her father after her mother was imprisoned for prostitution and involvement with illegal drugs. Her mother was dying of AIDS while in prison. Unfortunately, Jane's father suffered from severe alcoholism and soon that resulted in him losing all of his parental rights. Child Protective Services subsequently placed Jane and her younger sister with their paternal grandmother.

Grandma was very strict with the girls, but also very loving. She made sure they attended a Catholic school, regular and frequent church services, spent quality time together, and did not associate with "trouble" of any form or fashion. Both girls were very successful academically. In fact, while living with grandma, Jane always made straight "A"s and never needed disciplining at home, in school, or elsewhere.

As Jane approached her teenage years, she began to feel the need for more companionship than just her Catholic school girlfriends. During the summer of Jane's twelfth year, John, aged 15 at the time, orchestrated meeting Jane in their neighborhood. He would frequently walk the neighborhood streets, passing by her grandma's house several times a day, and would often stop to flirt with Jane whenever she was outside.

John attended public school, if and when he chose to, which was rare. He was a severely troubled juvenile delinquent, a "conduct disordered" child who evaded conforming with laws, regulations, rules, and expected decorum whenever such restrictions didn't suit his needs or wishes. With respect to Jane, however, John could be a real charmer when it suited his desires.

Within one month of meeting John, Jane began failing some of her classes. Within two months, her attendance at school was rapidly declining. Several parent-teacher conferences were arranged with Jane and her grandma. Jane would apologize for her bad behavior and promise not to do it anymore, even though she knew she would as soon as she was back with John.

After one such parent-teacher conference, Jane did get an "A" on a piece for her creative writing class. It was about a mean old spinster, who kept a young girl captive and isolated in her shack, until a handsome young lumberjack came and rescued her by killing the spinster. Her teacher questioned the unusual, albeit familiar, paradigm of Jane's creative piece. Jane responded that she was just exploring her emotions through creative writing. Despite

Jane's evermore frequent delinquency, the piece was brushed off by Jane's teacher as just another stellar academic performance by Jane. During this time frame, the school staff viewed Jane as having some emotional and social difficulties related to her spurt of adolescent maturation. No recommendation or referral was made for mental health counseling.

Within a month after submitting the creative writing story about the lumberjack, and despite her grandmother's numerous and stern protestations, Jane completely dropped out of school. She moved in with John and his mother, and slept in John's bedroom. They were now spending all of their time together, much of which was consumed with unsafe sexual activities. John continued manipulating Jane away from her family and friends and into isolation with him. Just before school was to break for Christmas recess, John initiated a conspiracy with Jane to kill her grandma. John was upset because Jane's grandma didn't want her to continue affiliating with him, did not want her living in John's house, and most certainly did not want her engaging in sex with him.

On the Friday after Christmas, while John's mother continued her daily routine of drinking, smoking, watching TV incessantly, and hoarding cats, John and Jane executed their premeditated plan. They walked from John's house over to her grandma's house and rang the doorbell. When her grandma answered, Jane ran inside and grabbed her younger sister, restraining her away from her grandma and the front door. John quickly wrapped a heavy kite cord around her grandma's neck, killing her by strangulation and exsanguination. The murderous act was so severe that an enormous volume of blood soaked through much of the carpet in the living room.

In a preposterous attempt to hide the evidence, Jane and John cut out a 10'x10' piece from the center of that bloodied carpet, rolled up grandma's corpse in it, and then stuffed grandma in her rug cocoon into the trunk of her own car. John and Jane then took Jane's younger sister upstairs and put her in a bedroom. John boarded and nailed shut the door and all the windows of the bedroom to prevent the younger sister from escaping.

John and Jane took all of her grandma's cash, her rolled-up corpse, and her car on a spending spree, buying superfluous trinkets and a lot of pizza, and then spent the rest of the day bowling and eating hot dogs. Upon returning to her grandma's house, they proceeded to have repeated sex, specifically choosing to use her grandma's bed, thinking that Jane's sister was still secured in the upstairs bedroom John had nailed shut. However, unsuspected by both John and Jane, Jane's younger sister had managed to break out of her makeshift prison through the boarded up window and fled barefoot through the heavy snow to a nearby home for help. That neighbor called the police, and John and Jane were arrested shortly thereafter in their naked glory on grandma's bed.

John's mother was an uninvolved parent, who preferred watching television instead of engaging her son in meaningful and substantive conversation. She rarely attended parent-teacher conferences at John's school, almost never followed through with any of the school's recommendations, and even more rarely kept appointments with the principal regarding John's incessant delinquent misconduct.

The post-murder investigation revealed John's psychopathy. During the investigation at John's home, law enforcement found over 28 cat carcasses that were either buried in shallow graves or rotting on top of the earth around the yard. They had each been systematically tortured, by burning in a microwave oven repeatedly over an estimated six to eight weeks each, before they succumbed and another cat was selected to take their place. Remnants of burned cat hair and flesh were still in John's mother's microwave oven. These sadistic acts of animal torture indicated that John was practicing and perfecting his torture skills for about 3 to 4 years prior to murdering grandma. That means that John had started torturing animals between 11 and 12 years of age.

Additionally, and before killing grandma, John had set his mother's barn on fire three times since age 10, which had brought him to the attention of Family Court and law enforcement. Despite all efforts, no one succeeded at rehabilitating John. Because of his conduct, Family Court placed him with his father, who was living north of Albany, NY.

John was also a chronic bed wetter, which occurred almost every night. He would tell Jane that he enjoyed "water sports," as he called it, which meant he enjoyed urinating on other people. He groomed Jane to become his water sports recipient.

By the age of 11, John was meeting the classic triad of sociopathy, namely torturing animals, pyromania, and chronic bedwetting. In his pretrial interview, John told the forensic psychiatrist that when he was about 11 or 12 years old, and living with his biological father north of Albany, he had killed and dismembered his father's girlfriend. He further added that he buried the pieces of her corpse in various, disparate locations. Smiling incessantly from ear to ear, he reported this to the psychiatrist as if he were preparing to gleefully kill the psychiatrist using his perfected microwave oven torture technique. It was impossible to know if John was toying with the psychiatrist or being truthful.

Immediately after the interview, the psychiatrist did notify the authorities. The father's girlfriend had gone missing during the time John lived with his father. Police with cadaver dogs responded to the report from the psychiatrist but were unable to unearth any physical evidence of John's alleged, brutal claim.

Both Jane and John were charged with murder and tried as adults. They were found guilty and sentenced as juveniles in accordance with state law. Jane received a sentence of six to nine years, because she did not actually participate in the act of killing her grandma. The day after her arrest and confinement at the Juvenile Detention Center, Jane was once again a model citizen. She returned immediately to getting straight "A"s, never broke the detention center rules, and even tutored her fellow inmates. She never received any disciplinary infractions and served approximately seven years before being granted early parole with monitoring for her good behavior.

Upon her release, Jane called the prosecutor on her case to express her heartfelt remorse for what she had done, and also to thank him for getting her convicted and sent to juvenile detention, because that had turned her life around. She even wrote to her former school principal to apologize for her behavior during the last three months when she attended school.

John received a sentence of nine years to life, because he actually planned and executed the murder. The same psychiatrist testified in John's trial that he manifested many signs and symptoms of psychopathy even at the early age of 11 or 12, according to John's own reporting.

In New York State, a convicted criminal can earn early release after serving three quarters of their sentence with good behavior. At the time he started serving his time, John was a scrawny, small-statured, frail-looking boy. He ended up serving 20 years in prison, 11 years of which were added onto his original sentence for repeated episodes of serious misconduct and infractions of the rules during his incarceration. At the time of his release, John had grown into a formidable adult, weighing 253 pounds and reaching a height of 6'3. He was released on parole in January 2014 after serving twenty years in prison.

Six months after his release from prison, the same psychiatrist that had testified for the prosecution at John's trial received a telephone call from the New York State Police (NYSP) in Albany. The NYSP senior officer stated that two of his troopers had made a parole inspection that morning of John's apartment, which was about 4 miles away from the psychiatrist's office. The troopers discovered that John had wallpapered his apartment with newspaper clippings containing articles about other cases in which the psychiatrist had testified. He had also posted numerous photographs of the psychiatrist. Each picture and clipping had been covered with a red magic-marker "X" and the word "KILL." Extensive arrangements were made to protect the safety of the psychiatrist. The fact that these displays were inside John's apartment meant that they would be viewed as his expression of free speech and not a threat to the psychiatrist. Hence, John had not technically violated his parole.

CASE 2: SUICIDE EPIDEMIC AT A GRADE SCHOOL

During the 2016–2017 academic year, in a small, rural community along the Hudson River in New York State, a chain of events unfolded in one school district that shocked the entire region. Nine-year-old Boy A committed suicide by a gunshot wound to the head using a Walter PPK 9 mm semiautomatic pistol. A couple of weeks later, ten-year-old Boy B committed suicide by hanging with a belt suspended from a closet hook at home after kicking a step-stool out from under himself. About a month later, another ten-year-old, Boy C, committed suicide by a gunshot wound to the chest using an unsecured revolver from his father's bedside stand. A week later, an 11-year-old, Boy D, stood in front of his school with a loaded semiautomatic Glock 45 pointed at the side of his head while proclaiming his intense desire to die.

Boys A, B, and C had pronounced their intentions, but their proclamations had sadly fallen upon unbelieving ears. The community desperately wanted to believe that kids these ages don't commit suicide. Fortunately, a teacher of Boy D took his threats seriously and contacted the school district assistant superintendent, while she continued to engage the boy with compassion.

A couple of weeks earlier the assistant superintendent had attended a day-long training on the information contained in this book concerning DRA and threat assessments (TA). She used the skills she had learned from that training to engage the boy in an empathic dialogue. She also called the forensic psychiatrist that provided the seminar in order to obtain emergency guidance on how to safely handle the crisis at hand.

She told the psychiatrist that Boy D had just moved to this school district two weeks earlier. His father was in prison for several violent acts involving firearms. Prior to his incarceration, the father had amassed a substantial number and variety of semiautomatic and fully automatic weapons, hunting bows, and a variety of knives. He taught Boy D extensively in the use of firearms as well the other weapons, so much so that Boy D knew exactly how to commit murder and suicide with his dad's Glock 45 and his other weapons.

Boy D was a special needs child with cognitive and learning challenges apparent since birth. He struggled academically, and spoke with a lisp, for which he was constantly teased. Unfortunately, Boy D was being bullied from the very first day at his new school. He hadn't yet made any friends or acquaintances. He felt very isolated and alone with no one to turn to. On top of all that, his mother had to work three jobs just to feed, clothe, and shelter her two children. Thus, much of the care for the six-year-old younger brother fell upon Boy D.

The psychiatrist stayed on the phone with the assistant superintendent, walking her through what to say to Boy D, how to say it, and so on. The psychiatrist also called New York State Police, local law enforcement and the county mobile mental health team from another line, explained the situation and the urgent need for an onsite evaluation and possible transport to the nearest inpatient child and adolescent mental health hospital. Local law enforcement arrived on the scene within minutes. The officers had also received the same DRA training and engaged with Boy D accordingly.

In the meantime, the assistant superintendent had secured the boy's trust sufficiently that Boy D agreed that she could call his mother and informed her of the situation. The mother immediately left work and proceeded to the school. A friendly and respectful interaction between Boy D and the police officers quickly grew. This made Boy D feel sufficiently comfortable to put down the Glock and walk backward away from it as requested by the police so it could be safely secured.

Boy D, his mother, the officers, and the mobile mental health team subsequently proceeded to the boy's home. The mother allowed the police to remove all firearms from the home and secure them at the police station. A safety plan was negotiated by all involved that allowed Boy D to stay at home with his mother. Mental health practitioners, the police, and social services checked in with the family daily, making sure the boy remained safe. They also took necessary steps to make sure the family's needs were met with social and financial assistance from social services, mental health services, and the school. This allowed the mother to increase the amount of time at home with her children, and for Boy D to be frequently reassessed. The longer term plan was to keep Boy D at home the rest of this school year and during the next school year initiate phasing him into the school community with extra supports.

CASE 3: GRADUATING SENIOR THREATENS SHOOTING AT HIS HIGH SCHOOL

Sean was a high honors senior at Valley High School. He had never been in any kind of trouble in school or otherwise. He never even had a referral to the principal, been in detention, or subject to any other form of disciplinary action. He was well liked by his peers, and was very active in Scouts. His father was an Eagle Scout leader. He was very close to his family, which comprised his father, mother, and sister. He and his sister were enrolled in the same school and in the same grade. His sister was the top academic achiever every year in school and was believed to be graduating as valedictorian. Sean had been a high honors student every academic year.

Sean's father was a successful small-business owner of a firearms sales and service shop, where Sean enjoyed spending much of his free time. Besides being an Eagle Scout leader, Sean's father was very involved in supporting the community by donating both time and money to the community and its various charities. His mother was also a very engaged and supportive community member. The entire family, including Sean himself, was very well liked.

However, Sean had some personal struggles. His entire life he had stuttered, which caused him personal angst, emotional pain, and social stigma. He had many friends, many popular friends in fact, but he still felt insecure socially due largely to his stuttering. He played varsity sports and enjoyed spending time with fellow team mates, yet again always feeling inferior because of the stuttering.

Sean's passion outside of school was metal tooling. He had an incredible ability to study pictures of something and then recreate it from metal. It was an artistic gift for him, so much so that he wanted to continue with it as his profession by making custom firearms. One day Sean saw a ballpoint-pen-sized handgun online that shot live bullets by pulling on the pocket clip, which served as the trigger. After careful and detailed study, he manufactured several of these 007 masterpieces in his basement shop, and each worked with absolute precision. He even made bullets for these "ballpoint pen guns."

Four months away from his graduation with high honors, standing on the school's sports field, Sean broadcast a message to his friends that initially did not receive much of a response. He posted on social media, "I'm so tired of all this bullshit I'm coming to the school with my guns and you'll see what happens next" and included pictures of his "pen gun."

The social media network at the school failed to follow "If you see or hear something say something" protocol and failed to report this message. Fortunately, after about 30 minutes, the message and picture came up on a 14-year-old girl's phone, who immediately became the adult on campus. She went directly to her favorite and most trusted teacher to show her the message. She asked the teacher to keep her name private, which the teacher did, except for the required protocol of notifying the principal. The principle took appropriate action. What was it?

A chain of events were immediately initiated and put into action. No one was injured and Sean received the mental health attention that he needed. Unfortunately, because he made that "terroristic threat" online, he was arrested and charged. He chose to strike a deal with the FBI and the federal prosecutor to serve three years in federal prison.

CASE 4: DEFINITELY NOT THE PERFECT PICTURE

Steven and his girlfriend, Suzie, live in a small town, where keeping close relationships with the family is preferred. Suzie had recently moved there to start a new life free of drinking and drugs. These close-knit towns are somewhat common in the area where they live. They're called "Onion Towns" by the inhabitants to reflect the underlying nature of the preferred inbred genetic pool. Although Steven and Suzie are not related to one another, they fall madly in love, and their passion produces a beautiful daughter, Sarah. As Sarah grows up, the relationship between Steven and Suzie sours. They split, and Sarah is placed with her mom but visits her dad regularly.

During the time period that follows, Sarah talks a lot at school with her peers about her newly kindled love relationship with a much older guy, who is teaching her grownup stuff, like how to use guns and rifles. She proclaims that she finds "DILFs" (Daddies I'd like to **ck) to be very hot. Word of this quickly spreads around her school, but it's written off as "just ridiculous teen-age fantasies." No one actually talks with Sarah about her creative writing subject matter, which has also become her primary subject in conversations with her peers. No one at school takes the time to engage Sarah in substantive conversation to explore her social and emotional condition as it relates to what she is proclaiming to her classmates.

When Sarah reaches the age of fifteen, she is showing physical maturation. She and her biological dad, Steven, grow closer. Soon thereafter, they each secretly proclaim their romantic love for one another. Nine months later, Sarah delivers a beautiful baby girl. Steven is the biological father of the baby. Sarah and her dad forge a marriage license application together, and father and daughter become husband and wife.

This incestuous relationship is kept hidden from Sarah's school, although her grades are falling at an alarming rate and her peers are spreading "rumors" about Sarah having married her "DILF." A parent-student-teacher conference is scheduled, and both Sarah and Steven, as daughter and father, feign everything is fine. "Sarah's just a normal teenage girl with some emerging adult fantasies. There are just a few issues with Sarah's mother, which we're all working on together in counseling as a family." Although uneasy with the situation, the school counselor and principal offer to be available should further support be desired by the family. Steven and Sarah thank the school for their concern.

Sarah and Steven raise their baby girl together as the now illegally married parental couple. Sarah drops out of school. When called in by the school about her lack of attendance, her father excuses her absenteeism by saying she has been very busy being a responsible mother for her child.

When the judge that married them based upon their forged marriage license application learns of this situation, he becomes enraged, orders their marriage nullified, orders Sarah into foster care with an older married couple, and orders Steven and Sarah to stay away from one another.

Love speaks louder than court orders. Steven secretly stalks Sarah. In the meantime, Sarah has not shown up in school over several weeks. She's been having sex with her adoptive father, and says she has fallen in love with him,

DILF #2. When Steven discovers this, he arranges to meet clandestinely with Sarah and ask her to come back home to rekindle their love relationship. Sarah agrees and the two return to Steven's home together and take up where they left off.

Sarah's adoptive father calls Sarah to find out why she hasn't been at home for several days. Sarah explains the situation to him, stating that she is in love with both Steven and him. Everyone agrees that all of them should meet up in order to figure out what to do.

They all meet at a remote location near the state border. The adoptive father is already waiting next to his car at the agreed-upon rendezvous site. Steven, Sarah, and their baby arrive, and Steven proceeds to get out of his truck. Before approaching her two DILFs, Sarah reaches into the baby's car seat and pulls out a semiautomatic handgun. She shoots and kills her adoptive father, then her biological father, Steven, then her infant baby, and finally kills herself with a gunshot to the head.

CASE 5: YET ANOTHER MALL SHOOTER

Toby is an overweight, Caucasian, 18-year-old young man with very low self-esteem and poor social skills. He's a loner and carries grudges about how he's been treated in school and by other peers. He has had emotional problems and counseling for many years. He is a victim of prolonged, severe, and chronic bullying.

Toby dropped out of high school before graduating and never got his GED. He lives with his parents in a very small home and does occasional manual labor for work. Since he was 13, Toby's parents have not entered his bedroom, which they claim was in order to respect Toby's privacy. Hence, they have not seen the memorial poster to the Columbine shooters, Dylan Klebold and Eric Harris, on their son's wall. They also have not seen Toby's journal containing page after page of enraged, hateful rants and threats written by their son.

One page in Toby's journal includes these entries: "4/20/xxxx will be redefining." "Doom at the school." "Be cruel to your school." "My will is your fate." "Suck my Glock." "The wolf within crawling out of my skin." "I'm the most cold blooded sonofabitch you'll ever meet." "I've waited my whole life for just this one day." "No hope = no fear."

No hope equals no fear is significant. People commit suicide because they feel helpless and hopeless about their situation changing. They pass into what is known clinically as the giving up–given up complex. Toby has given up and is ready to die for his revengeful plan.

In the upper left-hand corner of his Columbine memorial poster, which hangs on his bedroom wall, is pasted a local newspaper clipping with the title: "Police officers may begin patrolling the high school."

In early January following that newspaper article about police patrolling his former high school, Toby goes to a gun show in town, where he legally buys himself a Hesse-47 automatic assault rifle with no background check required. It is just a gun show, after all.

Given the fact that police will soon begin patrolling his high school, Toby quickly revises his plans—choosing an earlier date and a different site. On February 13, Toby drives over to the local Walmart, where he buys a dozen boxes of armor-piercing ammunition for his new rifle, along with enough magazines to hold all of those armor-piercing bullets. Then he drives over to the local mall just across the street from Walmart and parks outside the Best Buy entrance. He proceeds to load the magazines. He installs one magazine onto the Hesse-47 and stores many more in his cargo pant pockets. He gets out of his car to walk up to the Best Buy outdoor entrance.

Now, the mall is already open, including Best Buy. Toby could simply walk in with no problem. But that will not get him what he really wants. He desperately wants to be seen, to be the main attraction, to put on a show, and demonstrate how tough and cruel he can really be, and thereby achieve notoriety so no one will ever forget him. "Look how powerful and potent I really am! I'm not that timid, spineless, overweight, ignored, and unwanted guy everyone thinks I am." He is off the charts on Erikson's impotency scale.

Toby shoots several rounds through the Best Buy doors, breaking the glass panels, which shatter into hundreds of sharp shards that fall upon a newborn infant in a stroller being pushed by its teenage mother. He continues through Best Buy firing off more rounds, emptying more magazines. Many bullets pass through several rows of televisions and the heavy steel shelving spines that hold them, before they are stopped by yet another TV or yet another heavy steel shelving spine.

He then proceeds into the mall corridor, where he continues to empty more magazines. One older male shopper is hit. One bullet ricocheted off a metal pipe and hit a young active duty soldier in the knee, who was helping at the recruiting table. With his injured and bleeding leg, the soldier dragged himself across 25 feet of floor and into a women's dress store, where he camouflaged himself in a pile of dresses. However, the blood trail left behind I was quite visible.

The shooter stops once again to load a new magazine. That's when the mall security officers, who are off-duty police, tackle the shooter and secure him on the floor.

The young soldier is air evacuated to the Regional Trauma Center, where he immediately undergoes the first of numerous surgeries. He will never be able to serve in the military and feels "like my life is over." Today he remains disabled and unable to work.

The FBI agents want to perform the interview of the shooter, but first request guidance from the consulting forensic psychiatrist. They are told: "Pay special attention to the perpetrator's conduct while entering the Best Buy and while proceeding through the mall. He did this Gunsmoke Saloon guns ablazing, shooting through the doorway, made for Hollywood entrance. Why? Because he desperately wants to be noticed. No, he needs to be noticed. He has probably gone unnoticed, unseen his entire life. Even his parents don't see him, literally and figuratively. He's learned to see himself as a nothing, nobody in his own mind. In order to get him to open up and spill all the beans, notice him! Act very impressed." The psychiatrist also suggests that they "show excitement over his choice of weapon and shooting skills. Tell him how almost all of his bullets hit his intended targets. He won't know it's untrue, because he was too nervous and afraid to recall real facts. He'll believe whatever you say."

The two FBI agents get every detail from Toby in less than two hours. Toby tells the agents, "Thank god it was Sunday, because if it was Monday, it would've been a school." He takes a guilty plea to reckless endangerment, a charge that does not require proof of intent. But it bought Toby a 32-year sentence in a maximum security prison. He won't see an opportunity for parole until he's 50.

CASE 6: GOODBYE TEXT LETTER TO MY TEACHER

Dear Ms. Johnson, you are my most favorite teacher! I'm sure you know that by now. You have always made me feel worthwhile, even special in a way. Thank you for that. It always meant a lot to me.

I'm writing you this text, because my parents are fighting all the time—again. We all went for counseling, again, but it didn't work, again. Dad refuses to try anymore. He has decided to move out and go stay with his new squeeze, some floozy from across the river that I just cannot stand. She thinks we should be girlfriends, best friends even, but I can't stand her.

So mom and dad are finally going to get a divorce. And of course they both spend money like it's going out of style, when we have so many bills that need to be paid. Who's the responsible party in this family? Why does it always fall on my shoulders?

I'm feeling so depressed and unwanted. I feel like I should take this bottle of my mom's sleeping pills, along with her bottle of vodka, and permanently check out. I feel so helpless and hopeless. Nothing will ever get better. Most mornings it's hard for me to even get out of bed.

I don't know what else I can do. I feel paralyzed and unable to act, let alone act successfully. I did try suicide twice before, but only screwed it up and ended up sick as a dog in the emergency room, barfing for hours. Ooh, and I had to drink that god-awful charcoal stuff. Disgusting! I'm mostly afraid I won't do it right and then I'll be a vegetable for the rest of my sorry life. That would suck even more.

I know I need help. I want help in fact, but I'm afraid. I'm afraid I'll be locked up on a crazy ward somewhere and forgotten. My parents wouldn't even care.

By the way, I'm really sorry for my bad behavior in class the other day. Actually, the other 3 days. I just couldn't help it. This whole family mess has really gotten to me, and I just don't seem to be able to control my impulses anymore.

If there's any way you can help me, please call me. Please! I don't want to die, but I don't know what else I can do or who else I can turn to.

Very truly yours, Polly

Chapter 11

Lessons from Active Shooter Drills and Training

When an active shooter expands their desire to punish from an individual to a larger community, they are on a trajectory toward acting out their plan.

After each and every school shooting, school administrators across the nation all ponder the same question: "What do I need to do to prevent that from happening here?" This is a challenging question as most current administrators have academic degrees, certifications, and trainings that revolve around teaching and learning and leading others in educating young people. It is not in fields of safety and security.

Schools that employ SROs have a small sense of confidence in the security for the school but it is only a small degree of confidence. Many of the school shootings have found lists composed by the shooter(s) that denoted the SRO as a primary target. Of the numerous strategies offered by law enforcement and federal agencies, safety vestibules, threat assessment teams, and active shooter drills remain on the top of the lists for school safety. SROs consistently remain on the list as one strategy to utilize, but not one of the top five actions.

SROs are extremely valuable given their proactive approach toward providing a safe and secure school. They become a primary resource for students who may need a mentor that they feel comfortable confiding in. Developing this trust allows students an opportunity to have a positive role model in their lives. SROs do not police the hallways as guards; rather, they work daily with the students and staff in a positive manner to ensure a sense of communal safety.

Therefore, having an SRO or law enforcement walking through the schools provides a layer of safety and security, but it is not the only layer. When combined with proactive steps as outlined in this chapter, schools will be better equipped to both deter and manage an active shooter. Deterrence and management are critical components as 60% of active shooting incidents end before the arrival of law enforcement.

From Sandy Hook and numerous other school shootings much has been learned about state-of-the-art school safety and security measures. Safety vestibules, panic buttons, bullet-resistant glass, and solid core doors are excellent features that can be installed in schools across the nation at a low cost. To deter active shooters visible security will go a long way, and this includes vestibules and the presence of law enforcement. There are also other safety and prevention tactics that do not require funding that can be employed in schools. The only thing that must occur is a change in safety procedures by creating a new normal for schools.

First and foremost keep classroom doors closed and locked at all times. Under immediate stress and duress one of the first things to go are fine motor skills. Therefore there should never be a need to have to cross the room to go to a door to lock it. Knowing that there is a shooter in the hallway will further stifle the ability to act and walk toward the danger. This may initially be viewed as an inconvenience in the classroom, but it will go a long way in protecting students and staff should an attack ever occur.

Each school building should have a single point of entry for each building with no exceptions. This requires a safety vestibule, a type of holding tank. No one should be allowed out of the vestibule and into the school unless they were fully vetted. Parents, guardians, and siblings do not need access to the school building to drop off a forgotten book or lunch. Items may be left in the vestibule and retrieved by the monitor at a later time.

Driver's licenses and other forms of ID should be required for all individuals who request permission to enter the building. All staff assigned to the building should have ID badges that are worn at all times. These badges should clearly show a recent photo and the staff member's name. Staff members not assigned to the building must show their district ID badge and state the reason why they are requesting entrance to this building.

Driver's licenses and other forms of ID are required for all individuals who are not employed by the district. This includes delivery people, and community members. All visitors should sign in and out of the building. While in the building they should wear an ID that clearly denotes them as a visitor. People working the front desk (where visitors are allowed) should be staffed by those who know the students and community well. Never staff this position with a substitute.

Enforce a zero-tolerance policy regarding joking about school shootings and mass killings. After a majority of school shootings it was found that many active shooters engage in behaviors that signaled impending violence. To ensure the ability of staff and students to recognize this action as it is taking place, there cannot be a tolerance for kidding around about the POI. Once a student makes statements that are violent or do not seem normal it is critical that this information be shared immediately with school leaders. In turn the school leaders will conduct a DRA.

Establish, maintain, and promote a positive working relationship with your local policing agencies. Invite them to walk through your buildings daily, park in your lots when taking a break, and request their presence at all major events. The U.S. Department of Homeland Security (NTAC, 2013) offered the following advice: If the school does not have an SRO, encourage law enforcement to have a presence in your school. Invite them to speak in classes, offer them the opportunity to have lunch in the cafeteria, or provide space for them to complete administrative work. Their presence can equate to deterrence, and it may also provide opportunities for students to share thoughts and concerns in a safe environment.

Having a presence from law enforcement does not mean that there has to be an SRO. Working with the local police department, county and state policing agencies can help district's craft unique safety and security plans. Do not have a set schedule for these walk-throughs—the less routine the better. These walk-throughs should be encouraged even if the district employs an SRO—the more of a police presence, the greater the security.

Additionally, the policing agencies need to get to know the SRO so that they can work as a team should an issue arise. It is not beneficial to wait until an emergency is taking place to begin developing a positive relationship with policing agencies.

Schedule regular active shooter trainings for staff in every building in the school district, including the district office and transportation. Classrooms *are not* the only locations where active shooter incidents may occur. About 50% take place in classrooms and the other 50% occur in hallways, the cafeteria, and outside of the school. Safety actions need to become as reflexive as fire drills. We play how we train, so we need to train for all options.

Be sure to invite all first responders to these trainings as they need to practice with the actual buildings/structures. Along with training at the facility this is an opportunity for law enforcement and the school staff to get to know one another. When speaking with a NYS trooper about the response time to get to the school, the trooper allayed many fears when he stated: "There is a reason we have crash bars on the front of the cars. We are coming in if we have to take the wall down to do so." That comment brought tears to the eyes of those he was speaking to. They did not know each other, but this trooper made it clear that he was going to do all he could to protect them. This interaction would not have taken place had the active shooter drill not have occurred.

Active shooter training generally takes a full day. The training begins with a presentation about the training by law enforcement about the process, and reinforces the need to practice and follow all directions (there are trained instructors for this purpose). While the school staff are in the presentation, the first responders are getting a feel for the building and conducting their own training. Law enforcement will determine who will coordinate the command center and perimeter(s).

During the active shooter drills the staff will be assigned roles similar to their daily routines. While the drills take place, and there will be more than one, the staff will encounter different expectations. While waiting for first responders to arrive, school staff will undoubtedly have to make some life-and-death decisions. This is not something they are used to doing, so practicing this in a safe environment is critical for ensuring sound decision-making in the event of an actual active shooter. There are risks and options for how to respond, and these need to be communicated and practiced.

This may initially seem odd, but one major action that *must* take place during an active shooter training is the firing of blank rounds by law enforcement in various parts of the buildings. Hearing a gun fired outside is quite different from the sound it makes when fired inside a brick and mortar building. The age of the building, the amount of concrete, brick, carpeting, how many floors are in the building, and so on will result in different sounds. It is possible that a gun fired in the front foyer is not even heard on the second floor. A gun fired in the cafeteria may not be heard in the main office. Given this predicament, what then is the plan for when the first shot is heard? How will those who know that a shooter is in the school communicate this urgent knowledge to the rest of the school?

One school provided air horns to all of the classroom teachers and these are located by the classroom door. When gunshots are heard teachers will sound off their horn. As the horn is heard teachers in turn sound their horn. Consider it the same as the "wave" from a professional sports game, or as a new world version of alerting villages in medieval times by blowing through horns from atop hills and mountains. The horns will be going off around the building signifying a shooter is in the building. Other schools have provided each classroom teacher with the ability to make a school announcement using their school phones. One message is universally used that will be called over the intercom so that all can hear it. Find an option, train the staff, and implement it immediately.

An interesting fact is that in some buildings, especially older ones, when the gun was fired in the lobby it sounded like a bunch of books dropping to the floor. This is a critical realization for all staff. Moving forward they will choose to err on the side of caution and call a lockdown. Better to say I am sorry for interrupting the school day then to dismiss the noise that results in tragedy.

Another unique issue that has to be addressed is how will off-duty law enforcement identify themselves when responding to an active shooter at a school. It was clear that when that call goes out everyone hearing the call will be responding. The issue with different agencies responding, some in uniform and others not, is how law enforcement identify perpetrators from off-duty law enforcement. This is not something for the school safety protocol but it is something that the first responders need to be clear about. Thus, active shooter training affects both the school community and the first responders.

Be sure to plan time for teachers and staff to debrief and ask questions. Presenting and training is a large part of the security equation, but time has to be devoted to ensure internalization. In the classroom we call it checking for understanding and closure, so we need to practice what we preach with our staff.

Even though this chapter is entitled "Lessons from Active Shooter Drills and Training" it is worth noting the takeaways from the school shooting in Parkland, Florida, at Marjory Stoneman Douglas High School on February 14, 2018. The state of Florida created a commission to study the shooting in an effort to learn from the atrocity to prevent its recurrence.

1. First and foremost, maintaining secured entrances has to remain in place outside of the regular school day. Schools tend to be the focal pieces of the community and as such numerous activities take place at schools after the regular school day. Consequently, secured doors become unsecured as doors become propped open, single point of entry does not exist, and no one monitors the doors. Schools will always be the focal point for the community and keeping the school community safe requires maintaining safety protocols. Doors should never be propped open. Limit the number of doors that may be used for ingress and egress. Maintain monitoring of the doors as long as activity in the school is taking place.

2. Be sure to have an active shooter protocol. Every year all staff, as well as students, should receive training on this. Be clear with the protocol and call it what it is. Using colors or numbers will just cause confusion when the terror begins.

3. Have systems in place so that anyone, faculty, staff, or student, may enact an active shooter protocol. Everyone should be trained on how to access an all-call/loudspeaker/intercom system. This should be practiced throughout the year because fine motor skills are quickly lost during stress. Trying to make the all-call when shooting has begun does not generally equate with success. *You play how you train.*

4. To buy time for first responders to get to the school, it is important to have classrooms that can provide security. In Parkland a staff member died when they went into the hallway to lock the classroom door. Doors should be locked at all times so that the only action that may need to happen is to close the door. Better yet, during the school day doors should be locked and closed at all times.

   Take a look at your classroom doors. How much of the door is comprised of a window? Is it a hollow door or solid core door? Can you lock the door from inside the classroom? New technology allows for solid core doors and hardware that locks from the inside. Some states still require a minimum-sized glass window on all classroom doors. Be sure to purchase and install the highest rated bullet-resistant film for these windows. This door is often the only thing between an active shooter and your children. Don't skimp on the cost or technology. Schools need to buy time so that law enforcement can arrive.

5. Surveillance cameras are a school's best friend for overall safety and security. It is important to ensure that your system is up to date. Current cameras available today have high-definition imaging, night vision, and real-time imaging. The system in Parkland had a delay of over several minutes. First responders gained access to the cameras but were not aware of the delay. This caused quite an issue for law enforcement. Real-time and reliable information is critical.

6. It is important for school leaders to have a good working relationship with law enforcement. This relationship does not begin the day of the active shooting. It begins well before and should be maintained throughout the year, every year. Having such a relationship will allow for two-way communication with all students, and especially with students who exhibit qualities that cause concern for the student and the school community. Here is where the SRO plays a major role as their constant presence will help to build communication with school staff as well as with the students.

KEY IDEAS TO REMEMBER

Much can be learned from the debriefing that occurs after every incident of school shooting. Unfortunately, we have many sources of data for these events as they have been a bit too common over the past decade. George Santayane once said, "Those who cannot remember the past are condemned to repeat it." He stated that phrase in 1905, and in 2020 it is still very much relevant.

   Lessons learned from active shooters over the years prove one very important task is critical for school safety and security. Schools must conduct active shooter drills with their staff, annually if possible. Trainings must occur so that every building and possible active shooter location is practiced. We play how we train, so we need to ensure that when panic sets in and fine motor skills are lost, that we as educators can still protect our students and ourselves. This does not happen by just reading a book and talking about it, although those points do help. The drill has to be practiced.

Know too that when active shooter drills first begin there will be a lot of emotions and questions. Build in time to debrief and for talking about concerns and feelings. The staff need to internalize these trainings, so these days will be long and emotional.

Active shooter training takes time to plan for as it requires working in conjunction with first responders and numerous policing agencies. It is worth the time and angst for planning these days as the result is that all key stakeholders will know what is expected of them if an incident arises. They will have awareness of what options are available and they will know that there are going to be a lot of other people coming to their emergency. They are not alone. They are priority number one.

Active shooter training for students is very different, as it is less invasive. This type of training occurs by the way of lockdown drills. These drills are now required annually for schools across the nation. Required fire drills have been reduced and emergency drills such as lockdowns, lockouts, and evacuation drills have been added. For students, the key is to be out of the line of sight from the classroom door window. Students should take their backpacks with them to use as an additional shield should the shooter fire into the classroom. Remaining quiet is an important goal, and one that is understood to be the most difficult once an active shooter is in the building.

Students must move swiftly to get out of the line of sight and then barricade themselves with their backpacks, books, and/or desks. The teacher should help facilitate this and then remain calm and quiet with the students.

Along with thoroughly understanding what to do in the event of an active shooter, there are numerous actions districts can take to enhance school safety, many only costing a change in operating procedures. The top safety actions that need to occur include installation of a safety vestibule. No one should be admitted into the school building unless there is a very specific and validated reason for them. Anyone requesting permission to enter, even just to enter the vestibule, must have a valid photo id. As it currently stands in much of the public schools across the nation, it is far easier to gain entrance to a public school than an NFL stadium. This has to change.

Secondly, classroom doors must be closed and locked. Fine motor skills will be absent as soon as it is known that an active shooter is in the building. Students and staff have died in active shooter incidents because classroom doors were not locked. This just requires a change in the current operational procedures. Lock the doors!

Lastly, presence of law enforcement is quite a deterrent. This does not mean that the district must hire SROs. Law enforcement presence can be as simple as patrol officers including walking through the schools as part of their daily routine. An office can be provided with a phone and computer so that they can complete paperwork in the school. Officers may serve as guest speakers in classes and serve as chaperones. The possibilities are endless. What has to happen is the development of a relationship with all law enforcement agencies whose jurisdiction is within the school district. Develop these now so that people will recognize names and faces when an incident arises.

We play how we train. This phrase will never grow old as long as people consider shooting students in a school an option for showcasing their angst. Unfortunately, there will be another school shooting. The question is whether you are prepared for that. Do you know what to do, do you know what the students need to do? Do you know when and how law enforcement will arrive? Knowing the answers to these questions will allow for some peace of mind should an incident take place in your district, in your school, outside your classroom.

Chapter 12

Scenarios and Examples

Our greatest evils flow from ourselves.

—Jean-Jacques Rousseau

America bears witness to school shootings not just every year but practically on a monthly basis. Multiple mass shootings are all too common, with a few attacks occurring with multiple shooters involved. The rapidly escalating numbers of shootings and victims are staggering. In each of these violent instances, not only did the shooters proclaim specific information about their planned and impending school attacks, but other students, teachers, and family members also saw, heard, and/or knew one or more pieces of information about the impending attack before it was carried out. Had anyone reported what they knew or suspected they knew, and had there been a method for consolidating that data, those shootings may have been prevented.

Active shooters average four to five warning signs prior to enacting their plan. Warning signs can be a complete change in routine, temperament becoming more aggressive, work habits significantly declining, or postings on social media becoming more violent or demeaning, and at times there is the inclusion of alcohol or drug abuse. The warning signs were always present. Action on the part of noticing the changes in behavior did not always take place.

Unfortunately, people with knowledge of the warning signs and/or in positions of authority often didn't believe what the shooter(s) forewarned, denied to themselves that the warnings were potentially real, did not recognize the information as being known risk factors of a potentially impending violent act, and/or did not notify the appropriate skilled and trained authorities. This is not something to despair over, as most active shooters did not have any type of prior criminal history or history of violence. Therefore it is quite natural to be dismissive when actions and activities appear out of the norm. Given our new knowledge of what this change in behavior signifies, we can no longer be dismissive. Rather, we need to act.

Every citizen should know the four simple warning principles (see figure 12.1) and practice them without question.

If you see or hear something, say something! This is a twist on the more common "see something say something." The updated version includes hearing comments, podcasts, or any type of communication that causes you to take pause as the words are out of the norm.

Secondly, redundancy is required! Report what you saw or heard to a minimum of two people: start with your local law enforcement and also report it to someone of authority at the location/entity believed most likely to be the potential target/victim.

Check back with local law enforcement and a contact at the presumed target to ensure your concerns were heard and addressed. Keep in mind that

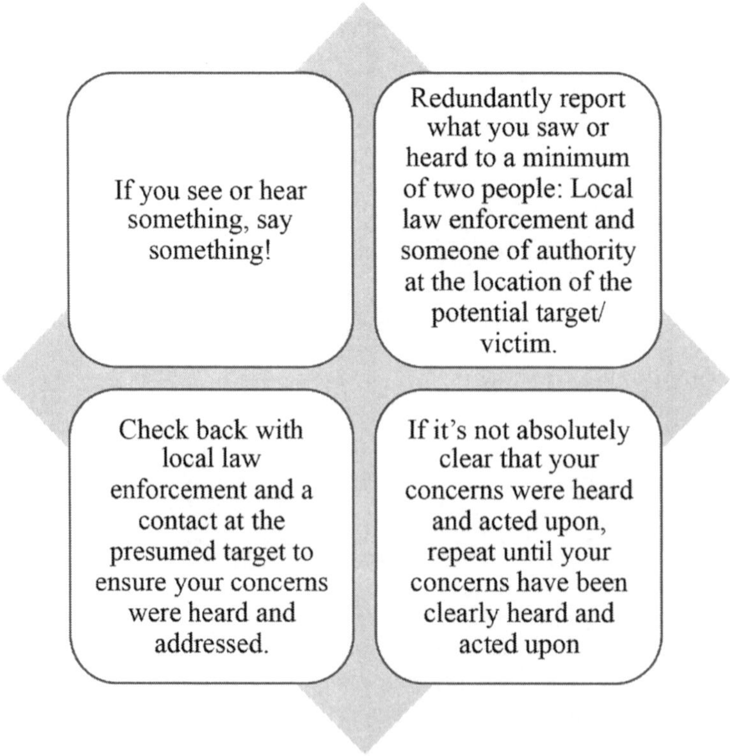

Figure 12.1   Four Warning Principles to Help Stave Off a Violent Act. *Source*: Self-Designed.

local law enforcement has built-in redundancy by virtue of jurisdictional overlap. For example, the State Police overlap with County Sheriff's Departments, which also overlap with Town and/or City Law Enforcement, and so on. When in doubt, rely on 911 to get your concerns to the appropriate agencies. That said, still call 911 back to verify that your report was entered into the system.

If it's not absolutely clear that your concerns were heard and acted upon, then repeat the steps until your concerns have been clearly heard and acted upon, and there is confirmation of your call and concern. Get the names of the people you spoke with if possible and write them down for reference. There should also be a call or file number generated regarding your call. Be sure to also write that number down.

These four principles are extremely important as illustrated in the following example that occurred prior to the shooting in Parkland Florida.

EXAMPLE 1

In months, days, and even hours prior to the Marjory Stoneman High School shooting in Parkland, Florida, several people witnessed concerning behaviors on the part of the shooter. Some of those people called those concerns into the FBI Regional Tip Line in Miami. That FBI Tip Line receives roughly over 5,000 calls on an average day. The good intentions of the callers were spot on, but the FBI simply could not sort through and prioritize all of those 5,000 tips in a day, let alone in hours or less. Those tips would have been much better placed to local law enforcement, from where officers would be immediately dispatched to a potential imminent threat in order to further assess, reassess, and formulate an appropriate plan of action and disposition, including immediately involving the FBI.

EXAMPLE 2

Within just a few days after the Parkland shooting, an engineer employed by Miami noticed that some alarming cracks were emerging in critical areas of a suspension walkway bridge at the International University of Miami. He immediately called in his concerning and relevant observations to the telephone number of the person he knew was responsible for following up on such concerns. Unfortunately, that person was away for a couple of days and no one else had been assigned the duty of taking those phone messages and making sure they were expeditiously acted upon. In the meantime, that bridge collapsed, injuring and killing several people. Those injuries and deaths could have been prevented if only communication redundancy had been built into the system and/or the reporting engineer had followed up on his concerns in short order.

Some of the principles were acted upon in the above examples, but the failure to follow up is of importance. Communication is the key to success. The same holds true when speaking about safety and security in our daily lives. The days of blissful innocence are no longer an option that we can engage in. Jean-Jacques Rousseau believed that man was born good and that society turns them into less civilized souls. Many people today fall into this belief that people are all good and civic minded, and do not tend to see the "bad" or "evil" in others. This is the paradigm in which humans function, and this same paradigm is often the cause of oversight or dismissiveness when someone acts or behaves out of the norm. It is time for the paradigm to change. *Failure to act causes the later need to react.*

Now is the time to see what you would do given the following situations. There really is no right or wrong answer, except that action must be the order of the day.

SCENARIO 1

John is your typical grade 10 boy who aspires to be on the varsity basketball team, and to help prepare he joins the cross country team in August to improve his cardio. Just as school is about to begin in the fall John's parents split up and his father moves out of the house. John, who previously was a straight A student struggles just to pass his classes. When speaking with the guidance counselor he shrugs it off, blaming new material and getting used to splitting his time between his mother and his father's homes.

As the first 5 weeks of school end, John is failing 3 courses and barely passing the others. As such he is removed from the cross country team where he was one of their top runners. In every meet that year he finished in the top three. After being removed from the team he was too embarrassed to hang out with his friends who are on the team and instead chooses to avoid the social scene.

Both parents tried to win John's positive attention and as such showered him with a computer, TV, and a host of computer games. John became addicted to playing online games which further isolated him from his peers and family. Soon John became friendly with online gamers and even began hanging out with one from a nearby town. His name is Sam. Sam loved to hunt and soon included John in on some hunting ventures. He had a couple guns whereas John had none, so he gave John one of his older guns.

John was enamored by the gun. He cleaned it almost daily at his father's home. His dad lived within walking distance from Sam. He stopped going to his mother's house, and if she pushed he would throw angry fits including a barrage of vulgar words. None of this was familiar to his mother as John was always polite and good natured.

When his mother addressed her concerns to John's father he dismissed it as her being jealous that John chose to be with his dad. However, his dad did question the change in behavior that included leaving childhood friends, poor academic performance, and a new passion for hunting. When looking at John's user history on the computer his father identified many gun sites, ammunition sites, war strategy sites, and lots of historical reviews of school shootings. When he directly confronted John about this, John stated that it was for a history project.

Your role in this is as a neighbor, whose son used to hang out daily with John. Your son, Tom, tells you almost daily about the bizarre behavior of John. You live next door to John's father and one day you choose to work from home. While looking out your window you can see directly into the backyard where John is target shooting. He has amassed a pile of various weapons and he is trying them all out. The target has the name of the high school written on it, the name of the guidance counselor, and a picture of his mother. What do you do?

SCENARIO 2

As a parent you often check the browser history of your grade 7 son as part of your agreement to give him a cell phone. While reviewing his Instagram and Snapchat accounts you notice that your son is frequently receiving podcasts and postings from another male. Upon further review you notice that this male appears to be a fellow student at the school who is voicing anger over not being popular, frustrated that the girls ignore him, and really upset about being passed over for a role in the school play.

Upon speaking to your son about this child, he is reticent about sharing any information about him. When pressed, he says, "You wouldn't like him, he says mean things, and is not very friendly." In turn you suggest that he not be friends with this child any more.

One week later your son comes home visibly upset. When asked why he is agitated he says that this boy was being mean to him because he couldn't be his friend. Your son is now a bit dejected and chooses to spend considerable amounts of time alone in his room. While searching his phone you find that he is looking up how to buy a gun, and what ammunition costs.

What do you do? Are you going to investigate this on your own? If not, who else will you share your concerns with? If your darkest fear is true, then what?

KEY IDEAS TO REMEMBER

What will be your 15 minutes in the limelight? For an active shooter it is not only the event itself but also the sequencing of events leading up to the shooting. Every active shooter made their intentions known. Whether anyone took them seriously is another story. Fact is they made it clear what they intended to do, and this was part of their time in the limelight.

It is far too easy to look back and critique others for not acting upon seeing or hearing information from the person who would soon become the active shooter. It is not for us to critique; rather, it is time for us to learn. We can no longer be dismissive of odd comments or actions. We have to acknowledge what we witnessed and then begin the actions to send the information to those who can best address the situation. Caught early enough, the comments and actions may easily be addressed through counseling. Addressing the issue toward the end may prevent a mass shooting. It is simple: action equates to prevention more often than not.

See something, say something is a phrase that became popular after the September 11 terror attacks. This phrase has since been slightly modified to *see or hear something, say something*. Only difference being the addition of hearing something, anything, that appears to be out of normal. This is the first of the Four Warning Principles.

Secondly, be sure to redundantly report your concern. Call and speak to more than one person, and make sure you record the date, time, person, and contact number for each phone call. The third principle is to check back with all the people you spoke to in principle #2. Mistakes happen, and things get missed. This is not one of those things that we can allow to go overlooked. Lastly, principle #4 is to repeat the first three principles until you know your concerns were heard and addressed. Maybe it turned out that it was not a credible threat. Or maybe it was credible, and they acted upon it thus preventing any aggressive action. Privacy laws will prevent them from providing you with details, but they can state if the concern was pushed up the chain of command.

The timing of following through on the Four Warning Principles is critical. As soon as you become concerned you need to act. The two scenarios presented in this chapter allow for an opportunity to determine when, how, and if action should be taken. Practicing scenarios often will allow for more options when an issue is at hand.

Chapter 13

What to Do When Confronted
by a Potential Attacker

*It is not the strongest of the species that survives, nor the most
intelligent, it is the one most adaptable to change.*

— Charles Darwin

At some point in our lives, a POI will stir up some very uncomfortable feelings. Anxiety, uncertainty, fear, an emerging or even imminent sense of
danger can cause anyone to panic. Consequently, one must know in the very
forefront of their mind what self-preservation options are available, which
ones they are able and willing to use, and from those options, which is the
best one for them to choose and adapt to that specific situation. There are
many instances where unarmed people successfully disrupted and prevented
an active shooter from causing harm. Both school staff and law enforcement
have the potential to deter a potential shooter based upon their personal
actions.

Everyone must personalize the options they have so that there is a comfort level for them when a choice needs to be made. The choice should be
made rationally, not emotionally. The optional plans available to school staff
and laymen will have specific requirements and guidelines to eliminate any
confusion. Plan details will be written in accordance with the organization's
master plan, policies, and procedures. The individual implementing the plan
will need to adapt to them in ways that allow them an acceptable level of
comfort in executing them. Professional law enforcement officers are unique
in that they are trained in clear-cut, precise, and specific protocols to be used.
So, where and how does one start?

Start with becoming very familiar with and memorizing these 7 mantras,
as illustrated in table 13.1.

Table 13.1   7 Steps for Surviving an Encounter with an Aggressor

Mantra #	Explanation
1	The very best laboratory for understanding human behavior and emotions is right inside each of us.
2	"I" statements are incredible lubricants for any conversation. Examples are "I'd like to hear what's bothering you," "I'd like to understand what made you feel so helpless and hopeless," and "I'd like to help you find a solution to this dilemma." Avoid using questions, commands, or the "W" words: who, where, what, when and why. They all sound and feel like an accusatory interrogation. Lastly, name calling is not appropriate at any time.
3	Hurt people hurt people! Words can be very hurtful. If the words used with the subject are hurtful to them, the risk of them harming you will rise.
4	Never ever play the sympathy card! It is infantilizing, irritating, and demeaning.
5	Breaking bread together is an incredible bonding opportunity.
6	Calmly tell the subject how frightened you are so that they can see past their own emotional storm and begin to see you.
7	If Mantras 1 through 6 fail to de-escalate the situation, flight and/or fight must be executed.

Self-Designed.

Mantra 1: The very best laboratory for understanding human behavior and emotions is right inside each of us.

Humans share around 99% of their DNA with other human beings. Therefore, practically speaking, most humans will have experienced, felt, thought, and done many of the very same things the POI has with respect to the current situation. One need not be a rocket scientist to correctly guess what the POI is probably experiencing emotionally, intellectually, or physically in response to the cause for their altered mood, thinking, and behavior.

Here's a tip: Pay close attention to what *you're feeling* in response to the totality of their presence, as this will likely be mirroring what they are really feeling inside. It's a universal and involuntary human response. Feel for it and use it! Avoid telling them what they feel. Instead help them open up and tell you.

Mantra 2: "I" statements are like invitations—incredible lubricants for any conversation.

Examples of "I" statements are "I'd like to understand what made you feel like taking your own life," or "I'd like to help you find a solution to this problem," or "I'd like to understand your perspective on what has caused you to be angry."

Avoid using questions, commands, or the "W" words: who, where, what, when and why. They all sound and feel like an accusatory interrogation. Name calling is not appropriate at any time.

The objective with "I" statements is to help the POI to comfortably reveal to you what is bothering them by your being receptive, open, nonthreatening, interested, and honest.

Never ever lie! Being lied to is one of the most common grievances and precipitators of resentments for everyone, especially POIs. If the POI asks how you feel, be honest in your response. If you're frightened say, "Yes, I am," or "Yes I am and thank you for asking," in a calm, controlled, and simple fashion, and with a tone that says you're grateful for their perception of how you feel. They may have already perceived how you feel anyway, which means they're really just testing your honesty. They're also likely to be an expert at detecting lying, because they've probably been lied to frequently by people who are supposed to care the most about them—a major source for some of the strongest grievances and resentments.

Mantra 3: Hurt people hurt people! If the words you use with the POI are hurtful to them, the risk of them harming you will rise.

Always treat them with respect, compassion, sensitivity, and concern. Never accuse the POI of wrongdoing. It will likely enrage them. When in a situation where the POI's emotions are growing stronger, do not threaten, demean, humiliate, bully, or use hateful speech. Learn the skill of not just demonstrating but actually feeling empathy. Empathy is the ability to step into someone else's shoes and appreciate what it must feel like for them from their perspective. Empathic statements should not be a declaration of how you think they feel but, rather, a statement of your appreciation of what they may be feeling.

For example, you observe that as the POI speaks about his girlfriend suddenly rejecting him and starting to date his former best friend, offer how that would make you feel as an "I" statement. Sharing an actual experience of your own in a generic form also works. For example: "I think I'm familiar with what you may be feeling. When I was your age, I was rejected by [my boyfriend], who didn't hesitate to latch onto a cheerleader instead of me. I felt devastated, hurt, angry." Rejection is a universal theme for all of us. Help the POI tell you their story, concerns, grievances, and resentments by being receptive, open, nonthreatening, interested, and *through the use of "I" statements.*

Mantra 4: Never ever play the sympathy card! It is infantilizing, irritating, and demeaning!

Playing the sympathy card suggests that the POI, in fact, is viewed as an infant or is acting like one. They may be, but pointing it out will not solidify your supportive and empathic relationship, which is what's required to create the desired safety zone. However, if they ask you if you think they're acting infantile, and you do, don't lie. Be truthful, but with a bland voice, like it's no big deal: "No problem. We all act infantile sometimes. In fact, I get accused of it more often than I'd like." The goal is to help them feel more akin to you, which will also help them feel more like an empowered, respected, and respectful person, who is capable of behaving in a mature fashion.

Mantra 5: Breaking bread together is an incredible bonding opportunity.

It cannot be overstated just how valuable breaking bread together can be when one finds oneself in a very threatening situation or even a standoff. It can take the wind out of the most stormy of sails. Be prepared to subtly and unnoticeably move the POI toward developing greater feelings of being respected, similar, and in the same social status. This is an exigent circumstance that may require you to cast some rigid laws, regulations, and rules aside in order to obtain a nonviolent, peaceful outcome.

For breaking bread together, always keep snacks and beverages in your pocket, your desk or somewhere nearby. Avoid having items containing caffeine or other stimulants, and "energy drinks" should not be used. However, if that's what is being strenuously demanded or is all that is available, use it anyway. It's still much better than nothing.

If you don't have any nearby, invite the POI to walk with you to the vending machines or the nearby convenience store to buy some for him. Talk as you walk and remember to use "I" statements. It creates a disarming condition. If the POI refuses to allow this, ask him if it's okay to request that your assistant retrieve the items to deliver to your location. If the POI agrees, make sure to tell the assistant to leave the items at a safe spot outside your location in order to avoid setting up a situation for the POI to obtain a hostage. Consider including some kind of code phrase or word in your master plan that messages anyone's assistant that a potentially dangerous situation is occurring and at what Cooper's level it is at. This construct can also be used if items requested by the POI are not available.

If items requested by the POI are, in fact, unavailable, simply brush the circumstance aside with a brief statement, such as "I just ran out yesterday evening and forgot to pick more up this morning." If the POI demands the desired product, follow the protocol above. Consider assuring them that you don't want them to mistake your following through with their request as a trick to sneak law enforcement into the situation. You will be the judge of whether this may be useful or not. If you choose to use such a statement, it will signal the POI that he has an opportunity to rethink his situation and plans. Again, this can advance an emerging bond.

Always have at least two each of sweet snacks, salty snacks, and beverages, as that will cover everyone's taste. The two sweet ones should differ from one another, as should the salty ones. Invite the POI to choose first and start munching, setting the stage for you to remark, for example, "Those cheesey doodles smell really good." This will be a subtle cue for the POI to offer to share. If they do share, that moment will become a significant turning point in the relationship, setting the stage for rapport to grow and for resentment to fade. You can also offer to share yours. And when the POI is finishing up the cheesey doodles, comment about them again. They may offer you a taste now, but if not, you've still made more headway toward a bond. You can work the evolving relationship even further by asking: How were they? Or, would you like something else? You should still have two snacks left and two more beverages. Weigh the pluses and minuses. If the POI asks for more and you have it, let them choose more. That will give you even more time to strengthen the bond and/or allow help to arrive.

Mantra 6: Calmly tell the POI how frightened you are so that they can see past their own emotional storm and begin to see you.

Let's say the POI has a gun pointed at you and he says the gun is loaded. That will frighten any of us. Communicating clearly and honestly with the POI is always the best option. First, calmly, slowly and without any sudden movements sit upright and still, slowly place your hands flat in your lap, open palms up and visible. It's harder to shoot a person that is entirely disarmed and unable to attack. Plus, your empty palms will allow the POI to relax more quickly.

Take a slow breath or two or three, and look the POI straight in the eye. Maintain your eye contact and blandly say something like:

- "I'm feeling very frightened right now."
- "I'd feel much more able to listen carefully if the gun was pointed away from me."
- "I'd like to focus on just listening to you. That would be easier for me if the gun wasn't pointed at me."
- "I'd like to work together on what's happening in your life right now."
- "I'd like to work together on fixing what's caused you to feel this way."

If the POI does point the gun away from you, when you sense a rapport has started to develop, and he's becoming more relaxed, tell him you will keep your hands in your lap, palms up, and will not make any rapid movements. The gun will still be available for him to use, but it's much less likely an accidental discharge will occur. You will definitely feel and therefore appear more relaxed. The more you can relax and meaningfully engage the POI, the better for both of you.

Avoid assigning ownership of any *feelings or actions* to the POI, as they may be upset and angry over a perceived grievance belonging to someone else with whom they feel close or imagine they are close. Use statements like these:

"I don't believe it's ever too late to help another person," rather than, "I don't believe it's ever too late to help you."

"If I've caused hurt in any way, I'd like to make amends to those I've hurt," rather than, "If I've caused you hurt in any way, I'd like to make amends to you."

Mantra 7: If Mantras 1 through 6 fail to de-escalate the situation, flight and/or fight must be executed.

Most persons find flight an easy consideration, but it may not be the best plan for saving one's students or oneself. Fight may be a better option. This will be a decision you will have to make in an extremely difficult position. Many say, "I just don't have a violent bone in my body," or "I could never attack another person no matter who they're threatening." It's time to reconsider that position, because when the decision that needs to be made is flight or fight in order to save your kids, it will be your decision to make.

Imagine being the matriarch elephant of a large herd in the Ngorongoro Crater of Tanzania, who is responsible for the safety of all of her brothers, sisters, children, grandchildren, nieces, nephews, adopted orphans, and so on. The lives of 35 or more extended family members depend on their matriarch for their well-being and safety. If a human extends their head outside of their jeep on the road down into the crater, the matriarch elephant will perceive a threat to her herd, charge the jeep and even flip it over, risking her own life to protect and defend her family. One day you may need to be that matriarch.

Even NYSED regulations allow for physical assault if needed to defend oneself or one's students from physical harm. You have the right to defend yourself and your students. There are two very useful defense tools to consider that are nonlethal and physically safer options for the classroom or office: some form of a whip and some form of a narrow stick or small club. The end of a solid, 3 to 5 foot length of braided leather whip with 8 or 9 tails hanging off the end is a great defense tool. A cane made from bamboo is also very effective. Even when made of rubber, these defense tools can sufficiently stun a would-be attacker to allow for escape, activating an alarm, or snatching away their own weapon.

Hopefully, your schools will have SROs, who are trained law enforcement officers. They can also provide the school staff with hands-on training in this area of emergency defense. Other law enforcement agencies within your area, such as state police, sheriff's officers, and military veteran organizations, also have skills in nonlethal tactical engagement. Ask what you are allowed and not allowed to have and use in your classroom for emergency attack situations. It's better to be well prepared and not have to use injurious or lethal force if at all possible.

KEY IDEAS TO REMEMBER

A POI will stir up some very uncomfortable feelings. Anxiety, uncertainty, fear, or emerging sense of danger can cause anyone to panic. The optional plans available to school staff will have specific requirements and guidelines to eliminate any confusion. They will be written in accordance with the organization's master plan, policies, and procedures.

Mantra 1: The very best laboratory for understanding human behavior and emotions is right inside each of us. Pay attention to what *you're feeling* in response to the totality of the POIs presence. This is a human response, to mimic the feelings of others, and it is helps ease the situation.

Mantra 2: "I" statements are like invitations—incredible lubricants for any conversation.

Avoid using questions, commands, or the "W" words: who, where, what, when and why. They all sound and feel like an accusatory interrogation. Remain as calm as possible and be honest in your replies. The tone of your voice is equally important, and it should be one that recognizes their actions.

Mantra 3: Hurt people hurt people! If the words you use with the POI are hurtful to them, the risk of them harming you will rise. Never accuse them of wrongdoing as it will only aggravate them more. Empathic statements should not be a declaration of how you *think* they feel, but rather a statement of your appreciation *of what they may be feeling.*

Mantra 4: Never ever play the sympathy card! It is infantilizing, irritating, and demeaning!

Mantra 5: The value of breaking bread is worth the time it takes to create the opportunity. Any type of food that can be offered to share helps to take some of the anger and ire out of the situation. Even just a stick of gum is of value in this situation.

Mantra 6: Calmly tell the POI how frightened you are so that they can see past their own emotional storm and begin to see you. This mantra requires you to appear as nonthreatening and calm as possible. Speak clearly and honestly and be sure to look the POI in the eyes. They need confirmation that you hear and see them.

Mantra 7: If Mantras 1 through 6 fail to de-escalate the situation, flight and/or fight must be executed. When the decision that needs to be made is flight or fight it will be your decision to make. Look around your surroundings for any type of item that may be useful as a tool to defend yourself with. A cane, crutches, baseball bat, anything that might help you protect yourself and those around you. This requires thinking quickly and creatively.

It is worth taking note of the 7 mantras in case an aggressive situation should ever occur and you find yourself in the middle of it. Keeping calm, being honest, sharing food, speaking clearly, and being honest with yourself will help you survive the situation and walk away. Sometimes you may find that you have to fight, and at other times you have to take flight, and sometimes you will have to stay and engage in conversation until help arrives.

Chapter 14

Trauma & Trauma Systems Treatment

Trauma is the opposite of healing.

As noted in chapter 1, the Johns Hopkins Center for Safe and Healthy Schools has already announced it will address the trifecta of school safety concerns: trauma, bullying, and gun violence. This chapter will look briefly at trauma and trauma systems treatment.

Trauma is an extremely disturbing and deeply distressing experience. It is best defined as "the opposite of healing." It is an all too common experience, and children are especially vulnerable.

The things that can count as childhood trauma, called adverse childhood experiences, or ACEs, are vast. The Center for Disease Control (CDC) reports that more than half of adults have experienced at least one ACE, and more than 1 in 10 have been through at least 4 different forms of ACE. These childhood traumatic experiences have long lasting physical, emotional, and interpersonal abnormalities. Additionally, new traumatic experiences after childhood, such as with active duty military personnel or a parent eye witnessing a loved one's car accident, can precipitate or reignite the emotional and physical problems that developed from the childhood traumatic experience(s).

There is no minimum or maximum number of ACEs one must experience in order to accumulate lifelong difficulties. However, the more ACE experiences one has had, the greater the risk of cancer, heart disease, strokes, cerebrovascular disease, chronic respiratory illness, depressive disorders, smoking, alcohol use disorder, unemployment, and even being uninsured.

That said, many people do exist who have experienced four or more ACEs that have managed to be or become healthy, happy, and productive members of society. Hence, early recognition of trauma and the provision of interventions to provide the victim with the cognitive and emotional tools to overcome their trauma are critical.

Is there something we can do before the point where a DRA is needed? Is there anything better than BRGRs, CBRGRs, SAD PERSONS, and Mantras? Can we identify kids early on as being at risk for growing up with elevated dangerousness risk? Could we make enough difference early in their lives to mitigate or even eliminate their future risk of violence?

One must start with an index of suspicion for ACEs, and the bar for suspicion should be set very low. It's better to capture all the kids that have experienced ACEs and include a few kids that haven't than to set the bar too high and miss any of the children that have had ACEs.

Suspect trauma when the child has any of the experiences noted in figure 14.1.

If trauma is suspected, the next step is to look for a trauma system in the child.

Trauma system looks like this: When confronted by stressors or reminders of their trauma, the traumatized child shifts to "survival-in-the-moment" status. They do this because their social and/or care environment does not, or cannot, help them regulate their physical sensations, emotional feelings, and behavioral responses. One should first look at the child's tendency to have dramatic shifts in emotions and behaviors when confronted by the stressor or reminder of it. This is called a "survival-in-the-moment" response. Think of signs of an impending stimulus response in the trauma system as similar to an emotional seizure.

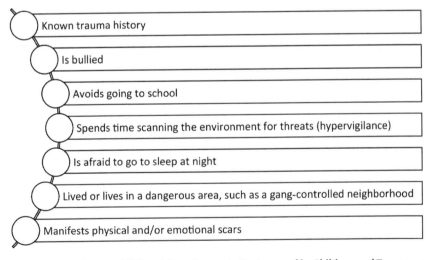

Figure 14.1   Adverse Childhood Experiences to Be Aware of in Children and Teenagers.
Source: Self-Designed.

Look for evidence of the following clues:

What was the child's trigger?
Where was the child introduced to the trigger?
When?
Why?
How?

When studying the child's possible trauma exposure, *safety is determined from the child's point of view*. Watch for patterns in the moment, patterns of links between the child's experience of a suspected threat in the present environment and evidence of transitioning to survival-in-the-moment status. Then answer the following questions:

When the child is exposed to stimulus Y, he responds with behavior Z.
This pattern can be understood through his past experience of X.

Determining past experience X is done by understanding his current stimulus experience, Y, and his current behavioral response, Z.

Think of signs of an impending stimulus response as analogous to an emotional seizure.

In order to detect an impending stimulus response, the observer must first observe and document how the child is in their normal state.

Next the observer will need to watch for signs of an emerging survival-in-the-moment state. The following observations will provide the observer with useful signs of an impending survival-in-the-moment shift. Those signs are observations of the following:

The child re-experiencing what seems similar to the trauma or threats of the trauma.

Revving, where the child's physical activities will increase in rapidity and intensity, such as tapping their foot, tapping their pencil, shaking one or more of their extremities, wringing their hands, throwing things, running out of the room, inability to respond to verbal interventions, and so on.

Changes in their speech and even ability to speak are common. The tone of their voice can change. Even partial or complete loss of ability to speak can occur. It seems as if they are ignoring you, but they're not. In order to defend against the perceived threat, their central nervous system has actually turned off the synapses that are needed to speak. They have been physiologically rendered temporarily mute.

This inhibition of normal speech or complete loss of speech capability is the peak of the "emotional seizure." This is where violence can and will occur.

The reconstituting phase follows after the "emotional seizure" phase. This is when the child gradually returns to their baseline state prior to exposure to the trigger. It is similar to the postictal phase following a grand mal seizure. It can be brief or prolonged.

Here is an example of a child who experienced multiple ACEs and the interventions that helped him to begin to overcome his trauma.

Jeffrey is a grade 6 boy. He has been having problems with his behavior at school. Jeffrey's paternal uncle, Harry, who is his legal guardian, has come in for several parent-teacher conferences and promised he would work with Jeffrey on improving his school conduct, but to no avail. Jeffrey's school behavior includes the following:

Scenario 1: Jeffrey, a normal and healthy-looking child steals a candy bar from a nearby store while walking to school. He takes out the candy bar in class and starts eating. His teacher requests, "Jeffrey, please put that away until after class." However, Jeffrey seems to ignore her request and just keeps eating, although a little faster.

His teacher isn't happy with Jeffrey's disobedience and commands, "Jeffrey! Don't make me send you to detention!"

In response to the teacher's threat, Jeffrey eats his candy more quickly and starts rapidly tapping his foot and pencil, remaining verbally unresponsive to her.

His teacher gets more upset with Jeffrey's persistent disobedience. She says, "If you keep pretending not to hear me, I'll have to immediately send you to the principal." Jeffrey suddenly springs from his desk, kicks his teacher in the leg as he runs past her out of the room.

Scenario 2: Jeffrey is in the cafeteria, lingering after all the other students have left. He politely asks the cafeteria counter worker for a second tray of food. She tells him that the cafeteria closed 5 minutes ago. Jeffrey asks again with a please, but she says no once again. Jeffrey's now visibly shaking. As his foot begins to tap, Jeffrey starts taking food from the counter top. The worker asks him rhetorically, "Didn't you hear me? I said the cafeteria is closed." There's no verbal response from Jeffrey, but he does start visibly shaking and again more rapidly tapping his foot. The cafeteria worker threatens to send him to the principal if he doesn't listen to her instructions and stop. Without speaking, Jeffrey throws his tray at her head and runs out of the school building, ignoring commands from a teacher in the hallway to stop.

Scenario 3: While walking down the hall, Jeffrey sees a half sandwich in another boy's backpack side pocket. He quickly snatches the half sandwich, unwraps it, and starts eating like he hasn't eaten in days. The assistant principal sees this and angrily confronts Jeffrey, demanding that he return the sandwich immediately. It's too late. Jeffrey has eaten the sandwich already and does not respond to the assistant principal at all. The assistant principal then demands loudly and firmly, "If you don't do what I say right now, I'll have to call your uncle, young man!" Jeffrey shoves the assistant principal forcefully and punches him in the face before he runs out of the building and off the campus.

You are the TST consultant. What is Jeffrey's current stimulus, what is his current response, and what clues do these provide regarding Jeffrey's original stimulus (ACE)?

Answer: In Scenario 1 Jeffrey was having issues with food. He behaved as if he was incredibly hungry, although he appeared healthy. He seemed so wrapped up in the candy it was as if he was just ignoring his teacher, although clearly his responses to her were evolving. He started showing evidence of revving by eating faster and rapidly tapping his pencil and foot. He also lacked verbal responsiveness to her. When she threatened to send him to the principal, Jeffrey sprang from his chair, assaulted the teacher and ran away.

In Scenario 2 Jeffrey lingered in the cafeteria after all other students had left. He wanted more food. He was polite about asking, but when the cafeteria refused, Jeffrey became visibly upset and was shaking. As his foot began to tap, he started taking food from the counter top. The cafeteria worker became verbally confrontational, to which Jeffrey did not verbally respond. Instead, he started visibly shaking and again more rapidly tapping his foot. When the cafeteria worker threatens to send him to the principal, and again without speaking, he verbally threw his tray at her head and runs out of the school building, seemingly ignoring commands from another teacher in the hallway to stop.

The three scenarios demonstrate that Jeffrey has issues with food, in particular the withholding of food. When denied access to food, he becomes nonverbal and starts revving, then runs away from the scene like he's frightened.

The ACE, or more accurately numerous ACEs, in Jeffrey's past is the reason. Both of his parents were severe drug and alcohol abusers, who had abused Jeffrey physically and emotionally. Child Protective Services eventually took Jeffrey away from his parents and placed him with his paternal uncle, Harry.

After he was removed from his parents' house and placed with his paternal uncle, the uncle proceeded to keep Jeffrey locked in the basement with no food or water, until he allowed his uncle to anally penetrate him. When he did, his uncle would reward him with food and drink, some supervised time out of his basement prison before returning Jeffrey to the basement. During his supervised time out of the basement, Jeffrey had to complete his cleaning chores of the entire house. The uncle threatened that if Jeffrey told anybody about the situation, he would torture Jeffrey to death.

When this paradigm was uncovered by the TST therapist working with the school, Jeffrey's uncle was arrested and convicted of his crimes. Jeffrey was placed with a very loving and caring family, who eventually adopted him. He remained in TST treatment through high school, making a remarkable recovery from most of his post-ACE behaviors and symptoms.

Early recognition of trauma and the provision of interventions to provide the victim with the cognitive and emotional tools to overcome their trauma are critical.

KEY IDEAS TO REMEMBER

Trauma is defined as the opposite of healing and is an extremely disturbing and deeply distressing experience. The things that can count as childhood trauma, called adverse childhood experiences, or ACEs, are vast.

The CDC reports that more than half of adults have experienced at least one ACE, and more than one in ten have been through at least four different forms of ACE. These childhood traumatic experiences have long lasting physical, emotional, and interpersonal sequelae. Additionally, new traumatic experiences after childhood, such as with active duty military personnel or a parent eye witnessing a loved one's car accident, can precipitate or reignite the emotional and physical problems that developed from the childhood traumatic experience(s).

There is no minimum or maximum number of ACEs one must experience in order to accumulate lifelong difficulties. However, the more ACE experiences one has had, the greater the risk of cancer, heart disease, strokes, cerebrovascular disease, chronic respiratory illness, depressive disorders, smoking, alcohol use disorder, unemployment, and even being uninsured.

Suspect trauma when the child has a known trauma history, avoids going to school, is bullied, spends time scanning the environment for threats (hypervigilance), is afraid to go to sleep at night, lived or lives in a dangerous area such as a gang-controlled neighborhood, and/or manifests physical and/or emotional scars.

If trauma is suspected, the next step is to look for a trauma system in the child. When confronted by stressors or reminders of their trauma, the traumatized child shifts to "survival-in-the-moment" status, because their social and/or care environment does not or cannot help them regulate their physical sensations, emotional feelings, and behavioral responses. One should first look for and at the child's tendency to have dramatic shifts in emotions and behaviors when confronted by the stressor or reminder of it, called a "survival-in-the-moment" response.

Look for evidence of the child's trigger, where, when, why and how the child was introduced to the trigger.

Remember when studying the child's possible trauma exposure, *safety is all determined from the child's point of view*. Watch for patterns in the moment, patterns of links between the child's experience of a suspected threat in the present environment and evidence of transitioning to survival-in-the-moment status.

Then determine the following: When the child is exposed to stimulus Y, he responds with behavior Z. This pattern can be understood through his past experience of X. Determining past experience X is done by understanding his current stimulus experience, Y, and his current behavioral response, Z.

Think of signs of an impending stimulus response as an "emotional seizure." In order to detect an impending stimulus response, the observer must first observe and document how the child is in their regulated (usual or normal) state.

Bibliography

ASIS International School Safety & Security Council. (2016). *Using Situational Awareness to Observe Pre-Attack Indicators*. Alexandria, VA: ASIS International.

Berlin, E. R. (2019, April 25). *New York State Safe Schools Task Force Recommendations [Letter to P-12 Education Committee]*. Albany, New York: NYS Education Department. Authorized by NYS Commissioner of Education, Mary Ellen Elia.

CLPS Consultancy Group, https://www.clpsconsultants.com.

"Gun Violence Archive." Gun Violence Archive. Accessed April 29, 2019. https://www.gunviolencearchive.org/charts-and-maps.

Humphrey, N., A. Kalambouka, M. Wigelsworth, A. Lendrum, J. Deighton, and M. Wolpert. (2011). "Measures of Social and Emotional Skills for Children and Young People: A Systematic Review." *Educational and Psychological Measurement* 71 no. 4: 617–637. Retrieved from https://doi.org/10.1177/0013164410382896.

Randall, E. D. (2019, April 29). "'Major Shortcomings' Found in NYS School Safety Actions." *OnBoard*. 6th edition, 20.

Silver, J., A. Simons, and S. Craun. (2018). A Study of the Pre-Attack Behaviors of Active Shooters in the United States Between 2000–2013. Federal Bureau of Investigations, U.S. Department of Justice, Washington, DC. 20535.

United States, United States Secret Service, National Threat Assessment Center (NTAC). (2000). *Enhancing School Safety Using a Threat Assessment Model* (p. 127). Washington, DC.: The Service.

About the Authors

Dr. Susan T. Vickers is a retired school superintendent who currently resides in Central New York. She has spent 30+ years in the field of public education, as a school superintendent, associate principal, and social studies teacher. At the State University of New York at Brockport she majored in Military History and Political Science while minoring in Math for her bachelor's degree and followed that with a master's in European History. Her administrative career began after earning a Certificate of Advanced Study at the State University of New York at Cortland in Educational Leadership. Ultimately, she earned a doctorate in Executive Leadership from St. John Fisher College in 2016. Throughout her career in education she was focused on doing what is in the best interests of the students while always ensuring a safe and supportive learning environment. The present title is Susan's first book.

Outside of working in the educational field, she is a budding pastry chef, enjoys coaching figure skating, and is a cycling enthusiast. She participates in the annual Tour de Cure Ride for Diabetes, and hopes to one day complete a century ride (100 miles). Her greatest accomplishment in cycling has been to complete 4 metric century (63 miles) rides.

Writing *School Safety: One Cheeseburger at a Time* with her friend, Dr. Kevin L. Smith, was a work of passion. She is committed to turning the tide against aggressive actions in schools. Columbine shocked us; Sandy Hook broke our hearts; and Parkland led to action. This book helps to keep the work going that was started by the students of Marjory Stoneman Douglas High School, or at the very least, this was the goal for her as she wrote the book.

Kevin L. Smith, M.D. is a Board Certified Forensic Psychiatrist with 40 years of experience in the field. He was born and raised in Denver Colorado. He majored in Chemistry and minored in Math at the University of Colorado

Boulder Campus, where he spent his summers volunteering as an Activities Aide at the Boulder Valley School for the Handicapable. He completed his senior year on a full-ride scholarship at the University of Regensburg in Germany. While there he tutored sciences and math at the Pindl Private School for Juvenile Delinquents, which he cherishes as one of his greatest lifetime experiences. After graduating college, he returned to Denver to complete his medical education at the University of Colorado. When his student loans maxed out, he obtained a grant from the Robert Wood Johnson Foundation to write a book titled "How to Finance a Medical and Dental Education," which the Foundation published. His research for that book made it clear that a military scholarship was his own best option to finish medical school.

The U.S Army chose Dr. Smith to serve at Walter Reed National Medical Center in Washington, D.C. for his Internal Medicine Internship and his Psychiatry Residency. There he had his first exposure to forensics as a fact witness in a father's mercy killing of his severely burned son, who was Dr. Smith's patient for an extended period of time. The outcome in that case was so disturbing to Dr. Smith that he felt unavoidably drawn into the forensic sciences.

After completing 10 years of military service, Dr. Smith settled in the Catskill Mountains of New York State. Here he built a reputation for turning decertified psychiatric programs into award winning services and for providing the courts with sound and objective expert testimony. The Supreme Court of The State of New York Appellate Division has twice cited Dr. Smith's forensic testimony in their decisions. In an infanticide case, the court upheld his testimony as more credible than the combined testimony of nine experts for the defense. In another murder case, his testimony was cited by the court in an extremely rare overturning of the lower court's verdict of guilty against a severely ill schizophrenic man, setting aside the jury's verdict and rendering in its place a judicial verdict of Not Guilty by Reason of Mental Disease or Defect.

Dr. Smith now lives in a 220 year-old historic stone house along the Hudson River in the Woodstock-Saugerties area of the Catskill Mountains. He enjoys hiking and camping with his dogs, kayaking, canoeing, mountain biking, snow skiing, the world class trout fishing in Roscoe, visiting the numerous famous historic sites of the Hudson Valley, occasional weekend excursions in Manhattan, and of course the plethora of arts and entertainment provided by world class professionals that come up to the area from metropolitan New York and/or live in this beautiful area.